ECG/EKG and Cardiac Conditions: Interpreting Key Disease Patterns

Noting Key ECG/EKG Signs of Heart Conditions for Easy Interpretation for All

By

DR. Joan HAMPTON

TABLE OF CONTENTS

Introduction
- Understanding the Role of ECG in Cardiac Diagnosis
- Basics of ECG Interpretation

Chapter 1: Myocardial Infarction
- ST-Segment Elevation Myocardial Infarction (STEMI)
- Non-ST-Segment Elevation Myocardial Infarction (NSTEMI)
- Q-Waves and T-Wave Changes

Chapter 2: Arrhythmias
- Atrial Fibrillation
- Ventricular Tachycardia
- Heart Blocks: First-Degree, Second-Degree, and Third-Degree
- Supraventricular Tachycardias

Chapter 3: Cardiomyopathies
- Hypertrophic Cardiomyopathy
- Dilated Cardiomyopathy
- Restrictive Cardiomyopathy

Chapter 4: Electrolyte Imbalance
- Hyperkalemia
- Hypokalemia
- Hypercalcemia
- Other Electrolyte Disturbances

Chapter 5: Structural Heart Diseases
- Atrial and Ventricular Hypertrophy

- Congenital Heart Defects
- Valvular Heart Diseases

Chapter 6: Other Cardiac Conditions
- Pericarditis
- Myocarditis
- Endocarditis
- Cardiac Tumors

Chapter 7: Pediatric Considerations
- Normal Variants in Pediatric ECGs
- Common Abnormalities in Pediatric ECGs

Conclusion and Clinical Applications
- Summary of Key Findings
- Practical Applications in Clinical Settings
- Further Reading and Resources

ECG Interpretation Exercises

Conclusion

INTRODUCTION

Welcome to "ECG/EKG and Cardiac Conditions: Interpreting Key Disease Patterns." We will explore the complex field of electrocardiography (ECG/EKG) interpretation in this extensive book, revealing the secrets surrounding the electrical signals produced by the heart and their importance in the diagnosis of cardiac disorders. This book is meant to be your reliable companion whether you're a medical student, a healthcare professional, or just a curious person wanting to learn more about the beats of the heart.

Understanding ECG/EKG tracings is akin to deciphering a complex language, with each waveform and interval holding crucial clues about the heart's function and potential abnormalities. Electrocardiography (ECG/EKG) is an essential, non-invasive tool used in the diagnosis, monitoring, and management of heart diseases. By recording the electrical activity of the heart from various angles, the ECG provides invaluable insights into the cardiac rhythm and structure, helping detect abnormalities that may indicate heart disease or conditions affecting cardiac function.

The ECG is important in the clinical setting for several reasons:

- **Detection of Cardiac Arrhythmias:** It helps in identifying abnormal heart rhythms, from common benign arrhythmias like premature beats to severe life-threatening ones such as ventricular fibrillation.

- **Diagnosis of Myocardial Infarction (Heart Attack):** ECG is critical in the early diagnosis and management of myocardial infarction. Specific ECG changes can indicate not only the presence of a heart attack but also its approximate age and the region of the heart affected.

- **Assessment of Cardiac Structure:** ECG can show signs of cardiac hypertrophy (enlargement of the heart), which may suggest long-standing hypertension or heart valve issues.
- **Monitoring the Effects of Drugs or Devices:** It is used to monitor the effects of certain cardiac medications or the functioning of devices like pacemakers.
- **Electrolyte Disturbances and Other Conditions:** Changes in the heart's electrical activity can also indicate electrolyte imbalances or other systemic issues such as thyroid disease.

For clinicians and healthcare providers, understanding how to read an ECG is like acquiring a fundamental language skill in medicine. Each segment and wave in an ECG tracing can reveal critical information about the electrical pathways and the health of the heart. By comparing these readings to normal ECG values and patterns, healthcare professionals can deduce various cardiac conditions, make timely decisions about emergency interventions, and plan long-term treatment strategies.

In the following chapters, we will explore these aspects in detail, providing a solid foundation for interpreting complex ECG tracings and applying this knowledge in real-world clinical scenarios.

From the ominous signs of myocardial infarction to the erratic beats of arrhythmias, we will explore a spectrum of cardiac abnormalities, shedding light on their distinctive ECG manifestations. Additionally, we'll go into the nuances of pediatric ECG interpretation and discuss practical applications of ECG analysis in real-world clinical scenarios.

As a foundational tool, the ECG is indispensable in both acute and chronic healthcare settings, providing immediate data that can be life-saving.

The Components of an ECG

- **P Wave:** This is the first short upward movement of the ECG tracing, representing atrial depolarization, or the spreading of the electrical impulse through the atria, which causes them to contract.

- **QRS Complex:** Following the P wave, this series of waves (a downward Q, a tall upward R, and a downward S) signifies ventricular depolarization, which leads to the contraction of the ventricles. The QRS complex is crucial in determining the ventricular health and function.

- **T Wave:** The upward curve following the QRS complex reflects ventricular repolarization, the process by which the ventricles reset electrically and prepare for the next beat.

- **U Wave:** Occasionally seen following the T wave, this small upward curve represents the repolarization of the Purkinje fibers. It's not always visible and can be influenced by various physiological and pathological conditions.

Important Intervals and Segments

- **PR Interval:** Measures the time from the beginning of the P wave to the start of the QRS complex, indicating the time the electrical impulse takes to travel from the atria to the ventricles.

- **ST Segment:** The flat segment between the end of the QRS complex and the start of the T wave; its analysis is crucial in diagnosing myocardial ischemia or infarction.

- **QT Interval:** This interval, spanning from the start of the QRS complex to the end of the T wave, represents the total time for ventricular depolarization and repolarization. Prolongation or shortening of this interval can be significant in various clinical conditions.

Reading an ECG
- **Rate:** Determining the heart rate from an ECG involves measuring the distance between R waves (RR interval) and calculating the rate based on this measurement.

- **Rhythm:** Identifying whether the heart rhythm is regular or irregular, which can be done by looking at the consistency of intervals between heartbeats.

- **Axis:** The mean direction of the electrical impulse during ventricular contraction, which can indicate the presence of conditions like ventricular hypertrophy or heart block.

- **Abnormalities:** Careful analysis of each component and interval for any deviation from normal can provide clues to various cardiac pathologies.

Through clear understanding and practice, these fundamentals of ECG interpretation allow healthcare professionals and students alike to identify normal and abnormal cardiac conditions effectively. As we progress in this book, each chapter will build upon these basics, exploring specific cardiac conditions and their distinctive ECG patterns in depth. This foundational knowledge is essential for accurate diagnosis and effective patient care.

Join me on this educative experience in the field of ECG/EKG interpretation, where every trace has a reason and every realization advances our understanding of how to diagnose the heart. As we commence our investigation, let us first review the fundamentals of interpreting an ECG trace and the significance of ECG interpretation.

CHAPTER ONE
Myocardial Infarction

Myocardial infarction (MI), also known as a heart attack, occurs when a part of the heart muscle doesn't receive enough blood flow. This lack of blood flow can lead to damage or death of that heart tissue. An electrocardiogram (ECG) is a vital tool in diagnosing and managing myocardial infarction, as specific changes in ECG patterns directly correlate with the type and severity of the attack. This chapter delves into the ECG manifestations of myocardial infarction, focusing on ST-Segment Elevation Myocardial Infarction (STEMI), Non-ST-Segment Elevation Myocardial Infarction (NSTEMI), and the implications of Q-waves and T-wave changes. Understanding these distinctions is crucial for timely and effective treatment, which can significantly impact patient outcomes.

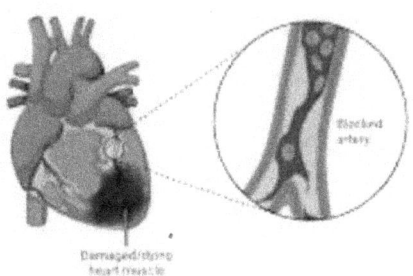

Fig 1.0: Myocardial

ECG changes specific to types of myocardial infarction provide clues about the location and extent of the infarction. For instance, STEMI and NSTEMI are diagnosed based on different ECG findings and represent different levels of coronary artery blockage. Additionally, the appearance of Q-waves and alterations in the T-wave can offer insights into the age and progression of the infarction. By examining these ECG patterns, healthcare providers can not only confirm the occurrence of a myocardial infarction but also implement the most appropriate therapeutic strategies. Let's explore each of these critical aspects in detail, beginning with ST-Segment Elevation Myocardial Infarction (STEMI).

ST-SEGMENT ELEVATION MYOCARDIAL INFARCTION (STEMI)

ST-Segment Elevation Myocardial Infarction (STEMI) is a severe form of heart attack that is identified by a distinctive elevation in the ST segment on an electrocardiogram (ECG). This type of myocardial infarction typically indicates a complete blockage of one or more coronary arteries, leading to a significant interruption of blood flow and oxygen to the heart muscle, which, if not promptly treated, can result in extensive heart muscle damage or death.

KEY ECG CHARACTERISTICS OF STEMI

- **ST-Segment Elevation:** The primary hallmark of a STEMI on an ECG is the elevation of the ST segment by more than 0.1 mV in two contiguous leads, which reflects acute injury to the heart muscle.

- **Location of the Elevation:** The location on the ECG where the ST segment elevation occurs can indicate the specific coronary artery that is blocked. For instance, elevation in leads V1 to V4 generally suggests a blockage in the left anterior descending artery, affecting the anterior part of the heart.

- **Concurrent Changes:** In addition to ST elevation, other ECG changes may include the development of new Q waves, which indicate necrosis of the heart muscle, and inversion of the T waves, which can occur as the condition progresses.

CLINICAL IMPLICATIONS

The prompt recognition and treatment of STEMI are critical. Treatment typically involves reperfusion therapy, which aims to restore blood flow to the affected area of the heart as quickly as possible. This is most commonly achieved through:

- **Thrombolytic Therapy:** Thrombolytic therapy, also known as fibrinolytic therapy. This treatment is used for certain conditions, including myocardial infarction (MI) (heart attack) and pulmonary embolism (blood clot in the lung). The administration of drugs that dissolve clots in the coronary arteries.

- **Percutaneous Coronary Intervention (PCI):** Percutaneous Coronary Intervention (PCI), commonly known as angioplasty. This procedure is used to treat coronary artery disease (CAD) and improve blood flow to the heart. A procedure that mechanically opens blocked arteries, often involving the placement of a stent.

MANAGEMENT STRATEGIES

Immediate management of STEMI also includes the administration of medications such as aspirin, anticoagulants, beta-blockers, and angiotensin-converting enzyme (ACE) inhibitors, which help reduce the workload on the heart and improve survival rates. Monitoring and management of cardiac risk factors and rehabilitation are also integral to improving outcomes after an initial STEMI event.

Understanding the ECG characteristics of STEMI and implementing quick and effective treatment not only saves lives but also significantly reduces the risk of complications and enhances the quality of life for survivors. In the following sections, we will discuss Non-ST-Segment Elevation Myocardial Infarction (NSTEMI) and how its presentation and management differ from STEMI.

NON-ST-SEGMENT ELEVATION MYOCARDIAL INFARCTION (NSTEMI)

Non-ST-Segment Elevation Myocardial Infarction (NSTEMI) represents a form of heart attack that, unlike STEMI, does not show the classic elevation of the ST segment on an electrocardiogram (ECG). NSTEMI typically results from a partial or temporary blockage of a coronary artery. This type of myocardial infarction is often less immediately dramatic than STEMI but still requires prompt medical attention to prevent further cardiac damage.

KEY ECG CHARACTERISTICS OF NSTEMI

- **Absence of ST-Segment Elevation:** In NSTEMI, the ST segment does not show significant elevation. However, subtle ECG changes such as ST-segment depression or dynamic T-wave inversion might be observed.

- **T-Wave Changes:** T-wave inversions or flattening in the ECG leads that reflect ischemic areas of the heart may occur.

- **Pathological Q Waves:** Unlike STEMI, NSTEMI may not show new Q waves, as the necrosis is not full thickness and may not be extensive enough to generate these markers.

CLINICAL IMPLICATIONS

Significant heart damage and subsequent cardiac events are still very likely with NSTEMI even though there isn't a noticeable ST-segment elevation. Assessment of cardiac biomarkers (e.g., troponin levels) indicative of myocardial injury is frequently part of the diagnostic procedure. Even in the absence of notable ECG abnormalities, elevated troponin levels can support the diagnosis of non-ST elevation myocardial infarction.

MANAGEMENT STRATEGIES

Management of NSTEMI typically involves a combination of medication and careful monitoring:

- **Medications:** Antiplatelet agents, anticoagulants, beta-blockers, ACE inhibitors, and statins are commonly used to manage and prevent further ischemia.

- **Risk Assessment:** NSTEMI patients are frequently put through a risk assessment process in order to ascertain whether invasive treatments such as coronary angiography are necessary, and if so, whether revascularization is feasible, depending on the severity and risk.

Early and aggressive management is crucial in NSTEMI to stabilize the patient, prevent further myocardial injury, and reduce the risk of progression to a more severe state or recurrent cardiac events. Follow-up care, including lifestyle modifications and possibly cardiac rehabilitation, plays a significant role in patient recovery and long-term heart health.

In the next section, we will delve into the specifics of Q-waves and T-wave changes, further exploring their significance in the context of myocardial infarction and their implications for diagnosis and management.

Q-WAVES AND T-WAVE CHANGES

Q-waves and T-wave changes are significant electrocardiographic findings that can provide crucial information about the presence, location, and timing of a myocardial infarction (MI). These ECG features help differentiate between acute and past infarctions and are essential in the ongoing assessment and management of patients with heart conditions.

Q-WAVES

Q-waves are the first negative deflections following the P-wave on an ECG and precede the R-wave. They are a normal part of a healthy ECG in certain leads. However, in the context of myocardial infarction, pathological Q-waves can develop:

Characteristics of Pathological Q-Waves:
- Wider than 0.04 seconds (one small box on ECG paper).
- Deeper than one-third the height of the ensuing R-wave in the same lead.
- Appear in leads corresponding to the location of myocardial damage.

→ **Implications:**
Pathological Q-waves suggest that there has been significant myocardial necrosis. They are typically seen after the acute phase of a myocardial infarction and can be permanent, serving as a marker of past MI. However, their absence does not exclude ongoing or previous myocardial ischemia.

T-WAVE CHANGES

T-wave changes, including inversion or flattening, are often seen in various stages of myocardial ischemia and infarction:

- **Dynamic T-Wave Inversions:** These occur during the acute phase of ischemia and are generally reversible if the ischemia is resolved promptly.

- **Persistent T-Wave Inversions:** May occur following an MI and can persist indefinitely as a sign of the changed ventricular repolarization resulting from scar tissue formation.

→ **Implications:**
T-wave inversions can indicate both acute and chronic heart issues. In acute settings, such as in NSTEMI or unstable angina, these changes necessitate immediate clinical attention to prevent further myocardial damage.

CLINICAL SIGNIFICANCE AND MANAGEMENT

- **Diagnosis**: Both Q-waves and T-wave changes require careful evaluation in conjunction with clinical findings and other diagnostic tests like cardiac biomarkers to diagnose and determine the extent of myocardial infarction.

- **Management:** The presence of Q-waves or T-wave changes can influence the management plan, including the urgency and type of intervention (medical management, coronary angiography, or revascularization procedures).

- **Prognostic Value:** Persistent Q-waves and T-wave abnormalities can provide insights into myocardial damage extent and are valuable for prognostic assessments, influencing long-term management strategies such as lifestyle changes, rehabilitation, and medication adjustments.

Comprehending the effects of Q-wave and T-wave alterations is essential for holistic heart care, as it allows medical professionals to customize treatments effectively and enhance patient results. When it comes to the diagnosis and treatment of cardiac patients, the ECG results are essential components.

CHAPTER TWO
Arrhythmias

Arrhythmias are disturbances in the normal rhythm of the heartbeat, characterized by irregularities in the heart's electrical impulses. These disruptions can lead to a wide range of cardiac abnormalities, from benign palpitations to life-threatening conditions. In this chapter, we explore several types of arrhythmias commonly encountered in clinical practice, including Atrial Fibrillation, Ventricular Tachycardia, Heart Blocks (including First-Degree, Second-Degree, and Third-Degree), and Supraventricular Tachycardias. Understanding the ECG manifestations and clinical implications of these arrhythmias is essential for accurate diagnosis and appropriate management.

INTRODUCTION TO ARRHYTHMIAS

The heart's rhythm is regulated by a precisely coordinated series of electrical impulses that initiate and coordinate each heartbeat. Disruptions to this intricate system can lead to irregular heart rhythms, known as arrhythmias. These abnormalities can arise from various underlying cardiac or non-cardiac conditions and can significantly impact cardiovascular health.

KEY FEATURES OF ARRHYTHMIAS

- **Atrial Fibrillation:** Characterized by rapid, irregular electrical activity in the atria, leading to an irregular and often rapid heartbeat.
- **Ventricular Tachycardia:** Involves rapid, abnormal electrical signals originating in the ventricles, potentially compromising cardiac output and leading to hemodynamic instability.
- **Heart Blocks:** Result from impaired conduction through the heart's electrical system, leading to delayed or blocked impulses between the atria and ventricles.
- **Supraventricular Tachycardias:** Include a variety of rapid heart rhythms originating above the ventricles, such as atrial flutter or paroxysmal supraventricular tachycardia (PSVT).

CLINICAL SIGNIFICANCE

Arrhythmias can have significant clinical implications, ranging from benign to life-threatening:

- **Symptoms:** Patients may experience palpitations, dizziness, chest pain, syncope (fainting), or even cardiac arrest, depending on the type and severity of the arrhythmia.

- **Complications:** Arrhythmias can lead to complications such as heart failure, stroke (in the case of atrial fibrillation), or sudden cardiac death (in the case of ventricular arrhythmias).

- **Treatment Challenges:** Effective management of arrhythmias often requires a multidisciplinary approach, including pharmacological interventions, electrical cardioversion, catheter ablation, or implantable devices like pacemakers or defibrillators.

IMPORTANCE OF ECG INTERPRETATION

An essential tool for identifying and treating arrhythmias is electrocardiography. Accurate interpretation of ECG tracings enables medical professionals to pinpoint the precise kind of arrhythmia, evaluate its severity, and choose the best course of action. The subsequent sections will delve into a detailed examination of each form of arrhythmia, emphasizing its unique electrocardiogram characteristics, clinical manifestation, and approaches for therapy. Let's start with one of the most frequent arrhythmias seen in clinical practice: atrial fibrillation.

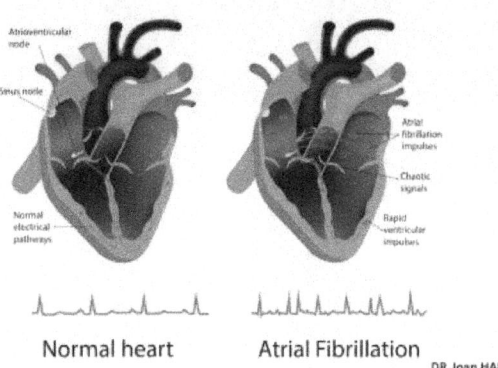

Fig 2.0: Heart Arrhythmia

ATRIAL FIBRILLATION (AFIB)

Atrial Fibrillation (AFib) is the most prevalent cardiac arrhythmia encountered in clinical practice, characterized by rapid, irregular electrical activity in the atria. This irregularity disrupts the coordination between the atria and ventricles, leading to an erratic and often rapid heartbeat. AFib is associated with an increased risk of stroke, heart failure, and other cardiovascular complications, making its diagnosis and management crucial in clinical care.

KEY FEATURES OF ATRIAL FIBRILLATION

Rapid, Irregular Heartbeat: Instead of the normal coordinated contraction of the atria and ventricles, AFib results in chaotic electrical signals, causing the atria to quiver or fibrillate.

- **Absence of P-Waves:** On an ECG, the absence of distinct P-waves is a hallmark feature of AFib. Instead, irregular, oscillating fibrillation waves (f-waves) are observed.

- **Irregular R-R Intervals:** The irregularity in ventricular response leads to irregular R-R intervals on the ECG tracing.

- **Variable Heart Rate:** The heart rate in AFib can be irregularly irregular, with rates ranging from normal to rapid, depending on factors such as autonomic tone, medications, and underlying cardiovascular conditions.

CLINICAL IMPLICATIONS

- **Increased Stroke Risk:** AFib is a major risk factor for ischemic stroke, primarily due to the formation of blood clots in the fibrillating atria, which can embolize to the brain.

- **Cardiovascular Complications:** AFib can contribute to the development of heart failure, particularly with a rapid ventricular response, leading to symptoms of dyspnea, fatigue, and exercise intolerance.

- **Impaired Quality of Life:** The symptoms associated with AFib, including palpitations, chest discomfort, and decreased exercise tolerance, can significantly impact patients' quality of life.

MANAGEMENT STRATEGIES

- **Rate Control vs. Rhythm Control:** Management of AFib involves strategies aimed at controlling heart rate and/or restoring normal sinus rhythm (rhythm control).

- **Anticoagulation Therapy:** Given the increased risk of stroke associated with AFib, anticoagulant medications (e.g., warfarin, direct oral anticoagulants) are often prescribed to reduce the risk of thromboembolic events.

- **Cardioversion:** Electrical or pharmacological cardioversion may be considered to restore normal sinus rhythm in symptomatic patients.

- **Ablation Therapy:** Catheter ablation procedures can be performed to target and eliminate the areas of aberrant electrical activity in the atria, particularly in cases of recurrent AFib refractory to medical therapy.

IMPORTANCE OF LONG-TERM MANAGEMENT

Long-term management of AFib involves a multidisciplinary approach, addressing risk factors such as hypertension, diabetes, and sleep apnea, which can exacerbate the arrhythmia. Lifestyle modifications, including regular exercise, weight management, and alcohol moderation, can also play a significant role in AFib management.

In summary, Atrial Fibrillation poses significant clinical challenges due to its association with stroke and other cardiovascular complications. Timely diagnosis, risk stratification, and appropriate management are essential for optimizing outcomes and improving the quality of life for patients with AFib.

VENTRICULAR TACHYCARDIA

Ventricular Tachycardia (VT) is a dangerous cardiac arrhythmia that is typified by frequent, swift electrical impulses that come from the ventricles and cause a rapid heartbeat. Hemodynamic instability can result from VT, and if left untreated, it can worsen into ventricular fibrillation, a potentially fatal arrhythmia linked to rapid heart death. For prompt action and better patient outcomes, it is essential to comprehend the ECG presentations, clinical consequences, and management techniques for VT.

KEY FEATURES OF VENTRICULAR TACHYCARDIA

- **Fast Heart Rate:** Ventricular tachycardia is defined as a heart rate exceeding 100 beats per minute, with the origin of the electrical impulse arising from the ventricles.

- **Broad QRS Complex:** On an ECG, VT is characterized by broad (>0.12 seconds) QRS complexes, indicating abnormal ventricular depolarization.

- **Regular Rhythm:** Unlike atrial fibrillation, which is irregularly irregular, VT typically presents with a regular rhythm.

- **Absence of P-Waves:** In VT, P-waves are often absent, as the electrical impulse originates from the ventricles rather than the atria.

CLINICAL IMPLICATIONS

- **Hemodynamic Instability:** Ventricular tachycardia can impair cardiac output, which can result in syncope, hypotension, disorientation, or even cardiac arrest.

- **Risk of Ventricular Fibrillation:** Sustained VT can deteriorate into ventricular fibrillation, a chaotic and life-threatening arrhythmia characterized by ineffective ventricular contractions and loss of consciousness.

- **Underlying Cardiac Disease:** VT often occurs in the setting of structural heart disease, such as coronary artery disease, myocardial infarction, cardiomyopathy, or electrolyte imbalances.

MANAGEMENT STRATEGIES

- **Immediate Cardioversion:** For hemodynamically unstable VT to return to normal sinus rhythm and avoid worsening into ventricular fibrillation, electrical cardioversion must be performed right away.

- **Antiarrhythmic Medications:** Pharmacological agents such as amiodarone, lidocaine, or procainamide may be used to terminate or prevent episodes of VT.

- **Implantable Cardioverter-Defibrillator (ICD):** Patients with a history of sustained VT or those at high risk of sudden cardiac death may benefit from the implantation of an ICD, which can deliver a shock to terminate ventricular arrhythmias.

- **Catheter Ablation:** In cases of recurrent or drug-refractory VT, catheter ablation procedures can be performed to target and eliminate the abnormal electrical pathways responsible for initiating and sustaining the arrhythmia.

IMPORTANCE OF LONG-TERM MONITORING

Patients with VT need to be closely monitored for an extended period of time in order to evaluate the effectiveness of treatment, find potential triggers or aggravating circumstances, and take care of underlying cardiac issues. In order to lower the chance of recurrence and enhance overall prognosis, lifestyle changes, adherence to drug regimens, and routine follow-up sessions are crucial aspects of VT therapy.

In summary, Ventricular Tachycardia poses significant clinical challenges due to its potential for hemodynamic instability and association with underlying cardiac pathology. Prompt recognition, appropriate management, and ongoing monitoring are essential for optimizing outcomes and reducing the risk of life-threatening arrhythmias in patients with VT.

HEART BLOCKS: FIRST-DEGREE, SECOND-DEGREE, AND THIRD-DEGREE

Heart blocks are irregularities in the electrical impulse conduction through the heart's conducting system that cause the signals between the ventricles and atria to be stopped or delayed from being transmitted. First-degree, second-degree, and third-degree heart blocks are the possible manifestations of these blockages; each has unique ECG characteristics and therapeutic consequences. Recognizing and treating possible consequences related to decreased cardiac conduction requires an understanding of the features and management of heart blockages.

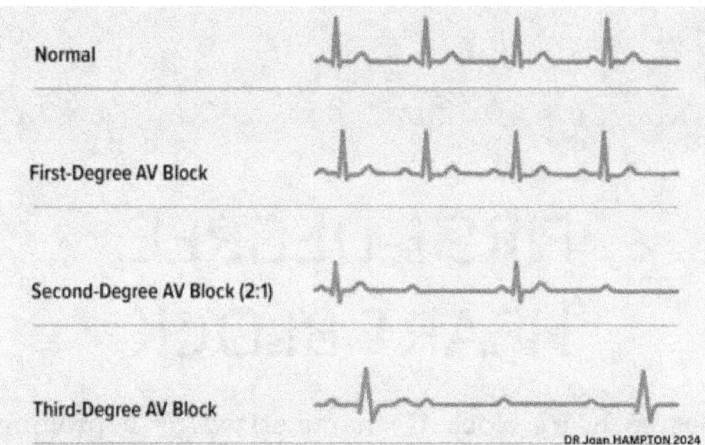

Fig 2.1: Heart Blocks

FIRST-DEGREE HEART BLOCK

First-degree heart block is characterized by a prolonged PR interval on the electrocardiogram (ECG), indicating a delay in the conduction of electrical impulses from the atria to the ventricles. Despite the delay, every atrial impulse is eventually conducted to the ventricles, resulting in a consistent 1:1 atrioventricular (AV) conduction ratio.

Key Features:
- **Prolonged PR Interval:** The PR interval, measured from the beginning of the P-wave to the beginning of the QRS complex, exceeds 0.20 seconds (five small squares) on the ECG.

- **Consistent 1:1 AV Conduction:** Despite the delay in conduction, every atrial impulse is eventually conducted to the ventricles, resulting in a normal QRS complex following each P-wave.

Clinical Implications:
First-degree heart block is often asymptomatic and benign, requiring no specific treatment.
It may be associated with underlying cardiac conditions such as myocarditis, digitalis toxicity, or degenerative changes in the conduction system.

SECOND-DEGREE HEART BLOCK

Second-degree heart block involves intermittent failure of atrial impulses to conduct to the ventricles, resulting in dropped or skipped beats. This condition is further classified into two types: Mobitz Type I (Wenckebach) and Mobitz Type II.

KEY FEATURES:

Wenckebach (Mobitz Type I):
- Progressive prolongation of the PR interval until a QRS complex is dropped.
- Typically observed in the setting of a normal QRS complex and a consistent pattern of conduction block.

Mobitz Type II:
- Consistent PR interval duration with occasional dropped QRS complexes.
- Often associated with more severe conduction system pathology and an increased risk of progression to complete heart block (third-degree AV block).

CLINICAL IMPLICATIONS:

Second-degree heart block may be asymptomatic or present with symptoms such as dizziness, syncope, or palpitations.

Mobitz Type II heart block is associated with a higher risk of progression to complete heart block and may require close monitoring and consideration for pacemaker implantation.

Third-Degree (Complete) Heart Block

Third-degree heart block, also known as complete heart block, involves complete dissociation between atrial and ventricular electrical activity, resulting in an independent rhythm for each chamber. The atria and ventricles beat at their intrinsic rates, leading to a slow and often irregular ventricular rhythm.

KEY FEATURES:

- **Complete Dissociation:** Atria and ventricles beat independently of each other, resulting in a slow and often irregular ventricular rhythm.

- **Atrial Rate > Ventricular Rate:** The atrial rate may be faster than the ventricular rate, especially in cases where an escape rhythm originates from the atria or junctional tissue.

CLINICAL IMPLICATIONS:

Third-degree heart block typically presents with symptoms of bradycardia, dizziness, syncope, or hemodynamic instability.

It is frequently required to implement a permanent pacemaker or temporarily pace in order to restore normal cardiac output and avoid consequences like abrupt cardiac arrest or heart failure.

MANAGEMENT STRATEGIES

- **First-Degree Heart Block:** Generally requires no specific treatment unless symptomatic or associated with an underlying condition requiring intervention.

- **Second-degree and Third-degree Heart Blocks:** May necessitate intervention with temporary pacing (e.g., transcutaneous or transvenous pacing) or permanent pacemaker implantation to restore normal cardiac rhythm and prevent adverse outcomes.

IMPORTANCE OF TIMELY INTERVENTION

Recognizing the type and severity of heart block is crucial for determining appropriate management strategies and preventing potential complications associated with impaired cardiac conduction. Close monitoring and collaboration between cardiology specialists and healthcare providers are essential for optimizing outcomes in patients with heartblocks.

SUPRAVENTRICULAR TACHYCARDIAS

A collection of cardiac arrhythmias that begin above the ventricles, usually in the atria or atrioventricular node, are referred to as supraventricular tachycardias (SVTs). Fast and consistent heart rates, frequently above 100 beats per minute, are the hallmark of these arrhythmias. The exact nature and underlying etiology of SVTs determine how they should be treated. They can show with a variety of clinical presentations and ECG abnormalities.

KEY FEATURES OF SUPRAVENTRICULAR TACHYCARDIAS

- **Origin Above the Ventricles:** SVTs originate from electrical pathways located above the ventricles, such as the atria or the atrioventricular node.

- **Regular Rhythm:** Unlike atrial fibrillation, which presents with irregularly irregular rhythms, SVTs typically exhibit a rapid but regular heartbeat on the ECG.

- **Normal QRS Complex:** In most cases of SVT, the QRS complex remains narrow (<0.12 seconds), indicating that the electrical impulse originates from within the normal conduction pathways of the heart.

- **Absence of P-Waves:** P-waves may be absent, distorted, or buried within the QRS complex due to the rapid atrial activity characteristic of SVTs.

COMMON TYPES OF SUPRAVENTRICULAR TACHYCARDIAS

- **Atrioventricular Nodal Reentrant Tachycardia (AVNRT):** AVNRT involves reentry pathways within the atrioventricular node, resulting in rapid and regular tachycardia episodes. It is one of the most common types of SVT and typically presents with a narrow QRS complex and absent or retrograde P-waves on the ECG.

- **Atrioventricular Reentrant Tachycardia (AVRT):** AVRT involves accessory pathways (e.g., Wolff-Parkinson-White syndrome) that bypass the normal conduction system, allowing for reentrant circuits between the atria and ventricles. AVRT may present with a narrow or wide QRS complex, depending on the presence of an accessory pathway.

- **Atrial Tachycardia:** Atrial tachycardia originates from abnormal automaticity or reentrant circuits within the atria, resulting in rapid atrial depolarization. It may present with a narrow or wide QRS complex on the ECG, depending on the site of origin and conduction properties.

CLINICAL IMPLICATIONS

- **Symptoms:** Patients with SVTs may experience palpitations, chest discomfort, dizziness, dyspnea, or syncope, depending on the rate and duration of the arrhythmia and individual patient factors.

- **Hemodynamic Effects:** SVTs can impair cardiac output and lead to symptoms of hemodynamic compromise, particularly in patients with underlying cardiovascular disease or structural heart abnormalities.

MANAGEMENT STRATEGIES

- **Vagal Maneuvers:** Techniques such as the Valsalva maneuver, carotid sinus massage, or diving reflex stimulation may be attempted to terminate SVT episodes by increasing vagal tone and slowing atrioventricular nodal conduction.

- **Pharmacological Therapy:** Antiarrhythmic medications, such as adenosine, beta-blockers, calcium channel blockers, or class IC antiarrhythmics, may be administered to terminate acute SVT episodes or prevent recurrences.

- **Cardioversion:** Electrical cardioversion may be necessary to terminate sustained or hemodynamically unstable SVT episodes, particularly when vagal maneuvers or pharmacological therapy are ineffective.

- **Catheter Ablation:** Radiofrequency catheter ablation is a curative treatment option for recurrent or refractory SVTs, targeting the abnormal electrical pathways responsible for arrhythmia initiation and maintenance.

IMPORTANCE OF COMPREHENSIVE EVALUATION

The management of SVTs requires a comprehensive evaluation, including clinical assessment, ECG interpretation, and consideration of potential triggers or underlying cardiac conditions. Tailored treatment strategies based on the specific type of SVT, patient symptoms, and risk factors are essential for optimizing outcomes and improving quality of life for individuals with supraventricular tachycardias.

CHAPTER THREE
Cardiomyopathies

Cardiomyopathies encompass a diverse group of heart muscle diseases characterized by structural and functional abnormalities of the myocardium, often leading to impaired cardiac function and heart failure. In this chapter, we explore three primary types of cardiomyopathies: Hypertrophic Cardiomyopathy, Dilated Cardiomyopathy, and Restrictive Cardiomyopathy. Comprehending the unique aetiology, pathophysiology, clinical presentations, and management techniques associated with each cardiomyopathy is crucial for precise diagnosis and efficacious therapeutic approaches.

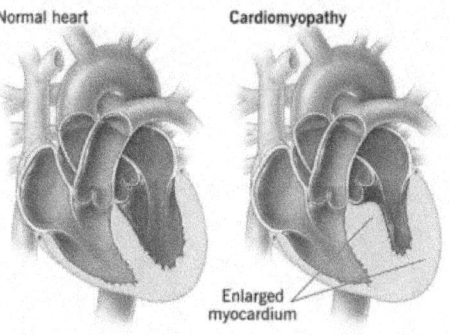

Fig 3.1: Cardiomyopathies

INTRODUCTION TO CARDIOMYOPATHIES

Cardiomyopathies represent a significant burden on global cardiovascular health, contributing to a range of clinical presentations, from asymptomatic myocardial dysfunction to life-threatening heart failure and sudden cardiac death. These conditions can result from genetic mutations, systemic diseases, environmental factors, or idiopathic causes, leading to structural remodeling and functional impairment of the heart muscle.

KEY FEATURES OF CARDIOMYOPATHIES

- **Structural Abnormalities:** Cardiomyopathies are characterized by structural alterations in the myocardium, including hypertrophy, dilation, fibrosis, or infiltration, which can impair cardiac contractility and relaxation.

- **Functional Impairment:** The structural abnormalities in cardiomyopathies lead to functional impairment of the heart, compromising its ability to pump blood effectively and meet the body's metabolic demands.

- **Clinical Heterogeneity:** Cardiomyopathies exhibit significant clinical heterogeneity, with varying degrees of severity, progression, and associated complications across different patient populations.

IMPORTANCE OF SUBCLASSIFICATION

Accurate diagnosis and focused treatment plans need the subclassification of cardiomyopathies according to morphological, functional, and etiological criteria. Accurate phenotypic characterization is crucial for clinical practice since every subtype of cardiomyopathy has unique clinical features, prognostic consequences, and treatment considerations.

In the following sections, we will delve into the pathophysiology, clinical manifestations, diagnostic evaluation, and management principles for three major types of cardiomyopathies: Hypertrophic Cardiomyopathy, Dilated Cardiomyopathy, and Restrictive Cardiomyopathy. By elucidating the unique characteristics of each cardiomyopathy subtype, we aim to provide clinicians with the knowledge and tools necessary to effectively diagnose, risk-stratify, and manage patients with these complex cardiac disorders. Let's start by learning about hypertrophic cardiomyopathy.

HYPERTROPHIC CARDIOMYOPATHY

A hereditary heart condition known as hypertrophic cardiomyopathy (HCM) is typified by aberrant myocardial thickness, or hypertrophy, especially in the left ventricle, without a known cause, such as aortic stenosis or hypertension. One of the most prevalent hereditary cardiac disorders, hypertrophic cardiomyopathy (HCM) affects people of all ages and can cause a variety of clinical symptoms, including asymptomatic hypertrophy, severe heart failure, and sudden cardiac death.

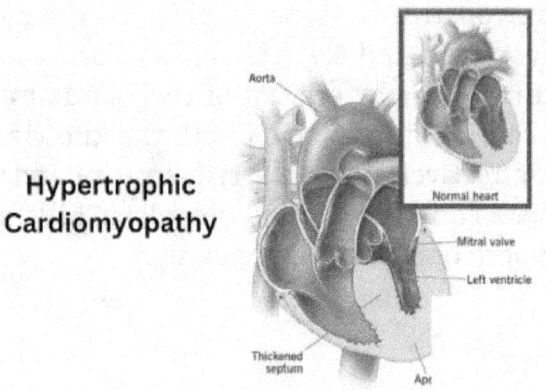

Fig 3.2: Hypertrophic Cardiomyopathy

KEY FEATURES OF HYPERTROPHIC CARDIOMYOPATHY

- **Myocardial Hypertrophy:** HCM is defined by unexplained left ventricular hypertrophy (LVH), often with asymmetric septal thickening, resulting in dynamic outflow tract obstruction and diastolic dysfunction.

- **Genetic Predisposition:** HCM is primarily caused by mutations in genes encoding sarcomeric proteins, such as myosin-binding protein C, beta-myosin heavy chain, and cardiac troponin, among others. These genetic mutations result in abnormal myocardial contraction and relaxation.

- **Clinical Heterogeneity:** The clinical presentation of HCM varies widely, from asymptomatic LVH detected incidentally on imaging studies to debilitating symptoms of heart failure, exertional dyspnea, chest pain, palpitations, and syncope.

DIAGNOSTIC EVALUATION

- **Echocardiography:** Transthoracic echocardiography is the primary imaging modality for diagnosing HCM, revealing the characteristic asymmetric septal hypertrophy, dynamic outflow tract obstruction, and mitral valve abnormalities.

- **Genetic Testing:** Genetic testing may be considered for individuals with a family history of HCM or when clinical suspicion is high. Identifying pathogenic mutations can help guide family screening and risk stratification.

- **Holter Monitoring and Exercise Testing:** Ambulatory electrocardiographic monitoring and exercise stress testing may be useful for assessing arrhythmias, including ventricular tachycardia and exercise-induced dynamic outflow tract obstruction.

MANAGEMENT STRATEGIES

- **Lifestyle Modifications:** Avoidance of vigorous physical activity and competitive sports is recommended for individuals with HCM to reduce the risk of sudden cardiac death and adverse cardiovascular events.

- **Medication Therapy:** Beta-blockers and calcium channel blockers are the mainstay of pharmacological therapy for symptom relief and prevention of dynamic outflow tract obstruction. Anticoagulation may be considered in select patients with atrial fibrillation or risk factors for thromboembolism.

- **Septal Reduction Therapy:** In patients with drug-refractory symptoms or severe outflow tract obstruction, septal reduction therapies such as septal myectomy or alcohol septal ablation may be considered to alleviate symptoms and improve hemodynamics.

- **Implantable Cardioverter-Defibrillator (ICD):** ICD implantation may be indicated for primary or secondary prevention of sudden cardiac death in high-risk individuals with HCM, particularly those with a history of sustained ventricular tachycardia or cardiac arrest.

IMPORTANCE OF LONG-TERM FOLLOW-UP

A multidisciplinary strategy combining cardiologists, genetic counselors, and other medical specialists is necessary for the long-term management of HCM. To track the course of the disease, evaluate the effectiveness of treatment, and spot potential side effects, comprehensive care must include routine clinical examinations, serial imaging scans, and genetic screening of at-risk family members. Healthcare professionals can enhance patient outcomes and quality of life for individuals with hypertrophic cardiomyopathy by instituting individualized management strategies that are tailored to each patient's unique risk profile and disease phenotype.

DILATED CARDIOMYOPATHY

Dilated Cardiomyopathy (DCM) is a heterogeneous myocardial disorder characterized by ventricular chamber enlargement and systolic dysfunction, leading to impaired cardiac contractility and heart failure. DCM is a common cause of heart failure and is associated with a wide range of etiologies, including genetic mutations, viral infections, toxic exposures, and autoimmune diseases.

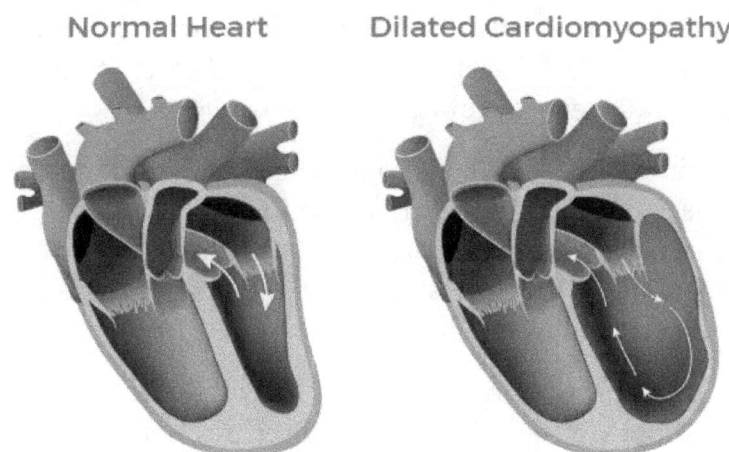

Fig 3.3: Comparison between Normal Heart and Dilated Heart

KEY FEATURES OF DILATED CARDIOMYOPATHY

- **Ventricular Dilatation:** DCM is characterized by progressive enlargement of the cardiac chambers, particularly the left ventricle, resulting in reduced myocardial wall thickness and increased chamber volume.

- **Systolic Dysfunction:** Impaired contractility of the myocardium leads to reduced left ventricular ejection fraction (LVEF), resulting in decreased cardiac output and heart failure symptoms.

- **Etiological Diversity:** DCM can have various underlying causes, including genetic mutations affecting sarcomeric or cytoskeletal proteins, viral myocarditis, autoimmune disorders, toxic exposures (e.g., alcohol, chemotherapy), and metabolic abnormalities.

Diagnostic Evaluation

- **Echocardiography:** Transthoracic echocardiography is the primary diagnostic modality for DCM, revealing left ventricular dilatation, reduced ejection fraction, and global hypokinesis of the myocardium.

- **Cardiac MRI:** Cardiac magnetic resonance imaging (MRI) may be used to assess myocardial tissue characteristics, identify myocardial inflammation or fibrosis, and evaluate for underlying etiologies such as myocarditis or sarcoidosis.

- **Genetic Testing:** Genetic testing may be considered in individuals with a family history of DCM or when clinical suspicion is high for an inherited cardiomyopathy. Identifying pathogenic mutations can inform prognosis, guide family screening, and influence management decisions.

MANAGEMENT STRATEGIES

- **Heart Failure Medications:** Pharmacological therapy for heart failure, including angiotensin-converting enzyme (ACE) inhibitors, angiotensin receptor blockers (ARBs), beta-blockers, and mineralocorticoid receptor antagonists (MRAs), is the cornerstone of DCM management. These medications improve symptoms, reduce morbidity and mortality, and slow disease progression.

- **Device Therapy:** Implantable cardioverter-defibrillators (ICDs) and cardiac resynchronization therapy (CRT) may be indicated in select patients with DCM and reduced ejection fraction to prevent sudden cardiac death and improve ventricular synchrony and function.

- **Lifestyle Modifications:** Lifestyle interventions, such as sodium restriction, fluid restriction, regular exercise within recommended limits, and avoidance of alcohol and illicit drugs, can help optimize heart failure management and improve outcomes.

- **Advanced Therapies:** In patients with refractory symptoms despite optimal medical therapy, advanced heart failure therapies such as heart transplantation, left ventricular assist device (LVAD) implantation, or cardiac regeneration therapies may be considered.

IMPORTANCE OF MULTIDISCIPLINARY CARE

Managing DCM requires a comprehensive, multidisciplinary approach involving cardiologists, heart failure specialists, genetic counselors, and other healthcare professionals. Regular clinical assessments, serial imaging studies, and close monitoring of heart failure symptoms and complications are essential for optimizing patient outcomes and quality of life. By addressing underlying etiologies, implementing evidence-based treatments, and providing ongoing support, healthcare providers can effectively manage Dilated Cardiomyopathy and improve the prognosis for affected individuals.

RESTRICTIVE CARDIOMYOPATHY

Restrictive Cardiomyopathy (RCM) is a rare but serious condition characterized by abnormal stiffness of the heart muscle (myocardium), leading to impaired ventricular filling and diastolic dysfunction. Unlike other types of cardiomyopathy, RCM is defined by restrictive filling patterns on echocardiography rather than significant ventricular hypertrophy or dilation. RCM can be idiopathic or secondary to various underlying causes, including infiltrative diseases, storage disorders, or endomyocardial fibrosis.

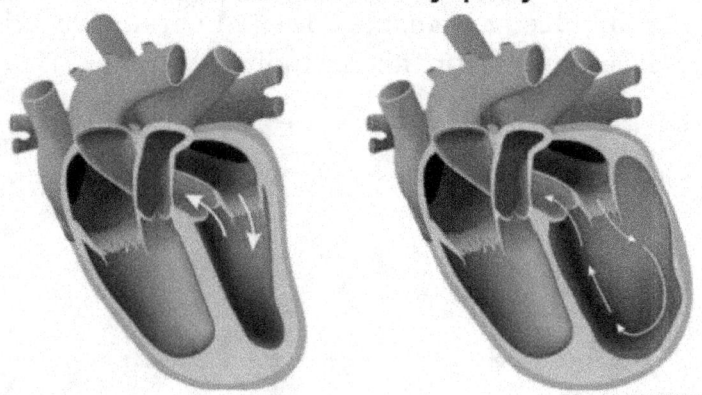

Fig 3.4: Restrictive Cardiomyopathy

UNDERSTANDING THE PATHOPHYSIOLOGY

In RCM, the myocardium becomes stiff and less compliant, hindering the ventricles' ability to relax and fill properly during diastole. This stiffness is often due to abnormal deposition of collagen or infiltration of the myocardium with substances such as amyloid protein, glycogen, or iron. As a result, ventricular filling pressures increase, leading to elevated atrial pressures, biatrial enlargement, and systemic congestion.

CLINICAL MANIFESTATIONS

- **Heart Failure Symptoms**: Patients with RCM may experience symptoms of heart failure, including dyspnea (shortness of breath), fatigue, orthopnea (difficulty breathing while lying flat), and peripheral edema (swelling of the legs).
- **Arrhythmias:** RCM is associated with an increased risk of arrhythmias, including atrial fibrillation, atrial flutter, and ventricular arrhythmias, which can further impair cardiac function and increase the risk of complications such as stroke or sudden cardiac death.
- **Systemic Congestion:** Increased filling pressures may cause systemic congestion, which may show up as peripheral edema, ascites (a buildup of fluid in the belly), or hepatomegaly.

DIAGNOSTIC EVALUATION

- **Echocardiography:** Transthoracic echocardiography is the primary imaging modality for diagnosing RCM, revealing characteristic findings such as biatrial enlargement, normal or small ventricular cavity size, thickened myocardium, and impaired ventricular filling with restrictive filling patterns.

- **Cardiac MRI:** Cardiac magnetic resonance imaging (MRI) may provide additional diagnostic information, particularly for assessing myocardial tissue characteristics and detecting underlying etiologies such as infiltrative diseases or storage disorders.

- **Endomyocardial Biopsy:** In cases where the underlying cause of RCM is unclear, endomyocardial biopsy may be performed to obtain tissue samples for histological analysis and guide specific treatment strategies.

TREATMENT STRATEGIES

- **Underlying Cause:** When the underlying cause of RCM is found, treatment focuses on treating it. This could entail particular treatments for infiltrative illnesses (such amyloidosis chemotherapy), enzyme replacement therapy for storage disorders, or endomyocardial fibrosis surgical excision.

- **Heart Failure Management:** Pharmacological therapy for heart failure, including diuretics, beta-blockers, and angiotensin-converting enzyme (ACE) inhibitors or angiotensin receptor blockers (ARBs), may be used to alleviate symptoms of congestion and optimize ventricular filling.

- **Arrhythmia Control:** In order to lower the chance of problems and enhance heart function generally, arrhythmias should be aggressively treated. Antiarrhythmic drugs, catheter ablation techniques, and the appropriate placement of pacemakers and defibrillators are a few examples of this.

Long-Term Outlook

The prognosis of RCM varies depending on the underlying cause, extent of myocardial fibrosis, and presence of complications such as arrhythmias or thromboembolic events. Close monitoring by a multidisciplinary team of cardiologists, heart failure specialists, and other healthcare providers is essential for optimizing treatment outcomes and improving quality of life for individuals with Restrictive Cardiomyopathy.

CHAPTER FOUR
Electrolyte Imbalance

Electrolytes play a vital role in maintaining the body's fluid balance, acid-base equilibrium, and neural and muscular function. Disruptions in electrolyte levels can have profound effects on various physiological processes, including cardiac rhythm, neuromuscular excitability, and renal function. In this chapter, we will explore common electrolyte imbalances encountered in clinical practice, including Hyperkalemia, Hypokalemia, Hypercalcemia, and other electrolyte disturbances. Understanding the causes, clinical manifestations, diagnostic evaluation, and management strategies for electrolyte imbalances is essential for providing optimal patient care and preventing potential complications.

INTRODUCTION TO ELECTROLYTE IMBALANCE

The maintenance of cellular membrane potential, osmotic balance, and neuromuscular excitability depend critically on electrolytes, which include sodium (Na+), potassium (K+), calcium (Ca2+), magnesium (Mg2+), chloride (Cl-), bicarbonate (HCO3-), and phosphate (PO4-). Electrolyte imbalances can be caused by a number of things, such as food consumption, kidney excretion, hormone regulation, drug use, and underlying medical disorders.

IMPORTANCE OF ELECTROLYTE HOMEOSTASIS

Maintaining electrolyte balance is essential for normal physiological function and overall health. Electrolytes regulate fluid distribution within the body, acid-base balance, and the function of vital organs such as the heart, brain, kidneys, and muscles. Even minor deviations from normal electrolyte levels can have significant clinical implications, ranging from mild symptoms to life-threatening complications.

The pathogenesis, clinical symptoms, diagnostic assessment, and therapy approaches for electrolyte disorders such as hyperkalemia, hypokalemia, and hypercalcemia will be covered in detail in the upcoming sections. Our objective is to equip healthcare professionals with the essential information and resources to identify, assess, and efficiently handle electrolyte disturbances in clinical practice by clarifying the mechanisms that underlie electrolyte imbalances and providing evidence-based approaches to their management. Let's look at hyperkalemia as our starting point.

HYPERKALEMIA

Hyperkalemia refers to elevated levels of potassium (K+) in the blood, typically defined as serum potassium concentrations exceeding 5.0 mmol/L. Hyperkalemia can arise from various factors, including impaired renal excretion, excessive potassium intake, cellular shifts of potassium from intracellular to extracellular compartments, or certain medications. Hyperkalemia is a potentially life-threatening condition that can lead to cardiac arrhythmias and cardiac arrest if left untreated.

UNDERSTANDING THE PATHOPHYSIOLOGY

The body tightly regulates potassium levels to maintain normal cellular function and membrane excitability. Under physiological conditions, potassium is predominantly located within cells, with only a small fraction present in the extracellular fluid. Disruptions in potassium homeostasis can occur due to impaired renal potassium excretion, such as in acute or chronic kidney disease, or increased potassium release from cells, as seen in conditions like rhabdomyolysis or tumor lysis syndrome.

CLINICAL MANIFESTATIONS

- **Cardiac Arrhythmias:** Hyperkalemia can lead to cardiac conduction abnormalities, including peaked T-waves, prolonged PR intervals, widened QRS complexes, and potentially life-threatening ventricular arrhythmias such as ventricular tachycardia or fibrillation.

- **Muscle Weakness:** Elevated potassium levels can impair neuromuscular excitability, leading to muscle weakness, paralysis, and potentially respiratory failure.

- **Nausea and Fatigue:** Patients with hyperkalemia may experience nonspecific symptoms such as nausea, fatigue, and malaise, particularly in cases of severe potassium elevation.

DIAGNOSTIC EVALUATION

- **Serum Potassium Levels:** Measurement of serum potassium concentrations is essential for diagnosing hyperkalemia. Levels exceeding 5.0 mmol/L are considered elevated.

- **Electrocardiography (ECG):** ECG findings may reveal characteristic changes associated with hyperkalemia, including peaked T-waves, prolonged PR intervals, widened QRS complexes, and eventually sine wave morphology in severe cases.

- **Renal Function Tests:** Assessment of renal function, including serum creatinine and estimated glomerular filtration rate (eGFR), is important for identifying underlying renal dysfunction contributing to hyperkalemia.

MANAGEMENT STRATEGIES

- **Calcium Gluconate or Calcium Chloride:** Intravenous administration of calcium gluconate or calcium chloride can stabilize cardiac cell membranes and antagonize the cardiac effects of hyperkalemia, particularly in the setting of severe or symptomatic hyperkalemia.

- **Insulin and Glucose:** Administration of insulin and glucose promotes intracellular shift of potassium ions, reducing serum potassium levels. Dextrose-containing solutions are often co-administered with insulin to prevent hypoglycemia.

- **Sodium Bicarbonate:** Intravenous sodium bicarbonate can help correct acidosis and promote potassium excretion via the kidneys, particularly in cases of metabolic acidosis associated with hyperkalemia.

- **Loop Diuretics:** Loop diuretics such as furosemide may enhance potassium excretion by increasing urinary potassium excretion, particularly in patients with preserved renal function.

IMPORTANCE OF MONITORING AND FOLLOW-UP

Close monitoring of serum potassium levels, electrocardiographic changes, and clinical symptoms is essential for assessing treatment response and guiding further management decisions. Long-term management of hyperkalemia focuses on identifying and addressing underlying causes, optimizing renal function, and minimizing risk factors for recurrent hyperkalemia. Collaborative care involving nephrologists, cardiologists, and other healthcare providers is crucial for optimizing outcomes and reducing the risk of complications associated with hyperkalemia.

HYPOKALEMIA

Hypokalemia refers to lower-than-normal levels of potassium (K+) in the blood, typically defined as serum potassium concentrations below 3.5 mmol/L. Hypokalemia can result from various factors, including inadequate potassium intake, increased potassium losses, or shifts of potassium from extracellular to intracellular compartments. Hypokalemia can have significant effects on neuromuscular and cardiovascular function, leading to symptoms ranging from mild weakness to life-threatening arrhythmias.

UNDERSTANDING THE PATHOPHYSIOLOGY

Potassium is an essential electrolyte involved in maintaining cellular membrane potential, neuromuscular excitability, and acid-base balance. Hypokalemia can occur due to increased renal losses, such as in cases of diuretic use, renal tubular disorders, or excessive urinary losses (e.g., from diuresis or polyuria). Other causes include gastrointestinal losses (e.g., vomiting, diarrhea, laxative abuse), inadequate dietary intake, or transcellular shifts of potassium into cells (e.g., alkalosis, insulin therapy).

CLINICAL MANIFESTATIONS

- **Muscle Weakness:** Hypokalemia can impair neuromuscular function, leading to muscle weakness, cramping, and fatigue. Severe hypokalemia may result in paralysis or rhabdomyolysis.

- **Cardiac Arrhythmias:** Potassium plays a crucial role in cardiac electrical conduction. Hypokalemia can predispose individuals to various cardiac arrhythmias, including ventricular ectopy, atrial fibrillation, and potentially life-threatening ventricular tachycardia or fibrillation.

- **Polyuria and Polydipsia:** In cases of renal potassium wasting, hypokalemia may be accompanied by increased urinary output (polyuria) and thirst (polydipsia) due to impaired renal concentrating ability.

DIAGNOSTIC EVALUATION

- **Serum Potassium Levels:** Measurement of serum potassium concentrations is essential for diagnosing hypokalemia. Levels below 3.5 mmol/L are indicative of hypokalemia.

- **Electrocardiography (ECG):** ECG findings may reveal characteristic changes associated with hypokalemia, including flattened or inverted T-waves, ST-segment depression, and prominent U-waves.

- **Renal Function Tests:** Assessment of renal function, urinary potassium excretion, and acid-base status can help identify underlying causes of hypokalemia, such as renal tubular disorders or metabolic alkalosis.

MANAGEMENT STRATEGIES

- **Potassium Supplementation:** Oral or intravenous potassium supplementation is the mainstay of treatment for hypokalemia, aiming to restore serum potassium levels to the normal range and alleviate associated symptoms. Potassium chloride is the preferred form of potassium replacement.

- **Identification and Correction of Underlying Causes:** Treatment of hypokalemia should include identification and correction of underlying factors contributing to potassium depletion, such as diuretic use, gastrointestinal losses, or metabolic alkalosis.

- **Monitoring Electrolytes and Cardiac Function:** Close monitoring of serum potassium levels, electrocardiographic changes, and clinical symptoms is essential during potassium replacement therapy to prevent overshooting serum potassium levels and minimize the risk of cardiac arrhythmias.

IMPORTANCE OF PREVENTIVE MEASURES

Preventing recurrent hypokalemia requires addressing underlying causes, optimizing potassium intake through diet or supplementation, and judicious use of medications that may exacerbate potassium depletion. Patients at risk of hypokalemia, such as those receiving diuretic therapy or with gastrointestinal disorders, should be closely monitored for signs and symptoms of potassium deficiency. Collaborative care involving healthcare providers from various specialties, including nephrology, cardiology, and internal medicine, is essential for optimizing management and preventing complications associated with hypokalemia

HYPERCALCEMIA

Hypercalcemia refers to elevated levels of calcium (Ca^{2+}) in the blood, typically defined as serum calcium concentrations exceeding 10.4 mg/dL (2.6 mmol/L). Hypercalcemia can result from various etiologies, including hyperparathyroidism, malignancy, excessive vitamin D intake, immobilization, and certain medications. Hypercalcemia can have significant effects on multiple organ systems, leading to symptoms ranging from mild gastrointestinal disturbances to severe neurologic and cardiac manifestations.

UNDERSTANDING THE PATHOPHYSIOLOGY

Calcium plays a crucial role in numerous physiological processes, including neuromuscular excitability, cardiac function, bone metabolism, and intracellular signaling. Hypercalcemia can occur due to increased bone resorption, decreased renal excretion, or extracellular shifts of calcium. The most common cause of hypercalcemia is primary hyperparathyroidism, characterized by excessive secretion of parathyroid hormone (PTH) leading to increased bone resorption and renal calcium reabsorption.

CLINICAL MANIFESTATIONS

- **Neuropsychiatric Symptoms:** Hypercalcemia can affect central nervous system function, leading to symptoms such as confusion, lethargy, depression, and impaired concentration.
- **Gastrointestinal Disturbances:** Patients with hypercalcemia may experience nausea, vomiting, constipation, and abdominal pain due to the effects of calcium on gastrointestinal motility and secretion.
- **Renal Symptoms:** Hypercalcemia can impair renal function, leading to polyuria, dehydration, and nephrolithiasis (kidney stones) due to increased urinary calcium excretion.

DIAGNOSTIC EVALUATION

- **Serum Calcium Levels:** Measurement of serum calcium concentrations is essential for diagnosing hypercalcemia. Levels exceeding 10.4 mg/dL are indicative of hypercalcemia.

- **Serum Parathyroid Hormone (PTH):** Assessment of serum PTH levels can help differentiate between hypercalcemia due to primary hyperparathyroidism (elevated or inappropriately normal PTH) and other causes such as malignancy or vitamin D toxicity (low or suppressed PTH).

- **Imaging Studies:** Radiographic imaging, such as skeletal survey, computed tomography (CT), or magnetic resonance imaging (MRI), may be indicated to evaluate for underlying causes of hypercalcemia, such as malignancy or hyperparathyroidism.

MANAGEMENT STRATEGIES

- **Hydration:** Intravenous hydration with isotonic saline is the initial treatment of choice for most patients with hypercalcemia, aiming to increase urinary calcium excretion and prevent dehydration.

- **Loop Diuretics:** Loop diuretics, such as furosemide, may be administered to promote urinary calcium excretion and facilitate fluid removal in patients with volume overload or severe hypercalcemia.

- **Bisphosphonates:** Intravenous bisphosphonates, such as pamidronate or zoledronic acid, are potent inhibitors of bone resorption and are commonly used for acute management of severe hypercalcemia, particularly in patients with malignancy-related hypercalcemia.

- **Calcitonin:** Calcitonin inhibits bone resorption and can provide rapid but short-lived reduction in serum calcium levels. It may be considered as adjunctive therapy in select cases of severe hypercalcemia.

IMPORTANCE OF UNDERLYING CAUSE IDENTIFICATION

The underlying cause of hypercalcemia should be found and managed, which may involve working with endocrinologists, oncologists, or other experts. Long-term management approaches could involve treating the underlying cancer, treating primary hyperparathyroidism surgically, or changing the drugs that cause hypercalcemia. For the purpose of evaluating the effectiveness of treatment and averting the recurrence of hypercalcemia and its related consequences, routine monitoring of serum calcium levels and clinical symptoms is crucial.

OTHER ELECTROLYTE DISTURBANCES

In addition to hyperkalemia, hypokalemia, and hypercalcemia, several other electrolyte disturbances can have significant clinical implications and require prompt recognition and management. These include abnormalities in sodium (Na+), magnesium (Mg2+), phosphate (PO4-), and chloride (Cl-) levels, each of which can affect various physiological processes and organ systems.

HYPONATREMIA

Hyponatremia refers to lower-than-normal levels of sodium in the blood, typically defined as serum sodium concentrations below 135 mmol/L. Hyponatremia can result from conditions such as volume depletion, syndrome of inappropriate antidiuretic hormone (SIADH) secretion, heart failure, liver cirrhosis, or certain medications. Symptoms of hyponatremia vary depending on the degree and rate of sodium decline and may include nausea, headache, confusion, seizures, and coma.

HYPOMAGNESEMIA

Lower-than-normal blood magnesium concentrations are known as hypomagnesemia, and are commonly described as serum magnesium concentrations less than 1.7 mg/dL (0.7 mmol/L). Inadequate intake, renal losses (such as diuretic use, renal tubular diseases), gastrointestinal losses (such as diarrhea, malabsorption), and drunkenness can all result in hypomagnesemia. Seizures, tremors, cramping in the muscles, and cardiac arrhythmias are some signs of hypomagnesemia.

HYPERPHOSPHATEMIA

Serum phosphate concentrations greater than 4.5 mg/dL (1.45 mmol/L) are commonly used to characterize hyperphosphatemia, which is defined as increased blood phosphate levels. Chronic kidney illness, hypoparathyroidism, high phosphate intake, and tumor lysis syndrome are a few disorders that can cause hyperphosphatemia. Even though hyperphosphatemia is frequently asymptomatic, over time it can cause consequences such renal osteodystrophy, metastatic calcifications, and cardiovascular disease.

HYPOCHLOREMIA

Hypochloremia refers to lower-than-normal levels of chloride in the blood, typically defined as serum chloride concentrations below 96 mmol/L. Hypochloremia can occur secondary to conditions such as vomiting, diarrhea, excessive sweating, metabolic alkalosis, or certain medications (e.g., diuretics). Symptoms of hypochloremia may include weakness, lethargy, muscle cramps, and metabolic alkalosis.

MANAGEMENT STRATEGIES

Management of other electrolyte disturbances involves identifying and addressing underlying causes, correcting electrolyte imbalances, and preventing complications associated with abnormal levels. Treatment may include fluid resuscitation, electrolyte replacement therapy, addressing the underlying medical condition, and discontinuing medications contributing to electrolyte abnormalities. Close monitoring of electrolyte levels, renal function, and clinical symptoms is essential for guiding management and optimizing patient outcomes.

Electrolyte disturbances can have profound effects on physiological function and clinical outcomes. Recognition of these disturbances, prompt diagnostic evaluation, and appropriate management are essential components of patient care. By understanding the pathophysiology, clinical manifestations, and management strategies for various electrolyte imbalances, healthcare providers can effectively identify and treat these conditions, ultimately improving patient outcomes and quality of life.

CHAPTER FIVE
Structural Heart Diseases

Structural heart diseases encompass a diverse group of conditions affecting the anatomy and function of the heart's chambers, valves, and supporting structures. These conditions can arise from congenital abnormalities, acquired disorders, or age-related degenerative changes, leading to impaired cardiac function and potential complications. In this chapter, we will explore various structural heart diseases, including atrial and ventricular hypertrophy, congenital heart defects, and valvular heart diseases. Understanding the pathophysiology, clinical manifestations, diagnostic evaluation, and management strategies for these conditions is essential for providing comprehensive care to affected individuals.

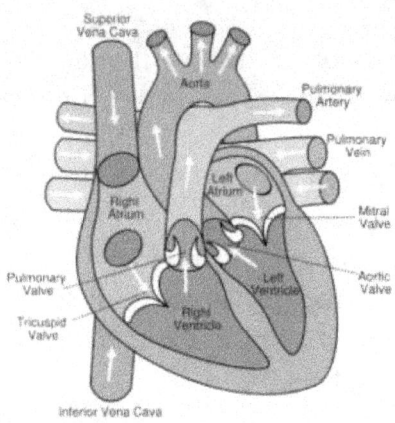

Fig 5.0: Structural Heart

INTRODUCTION TO STRUCTURAL HEART DISEASES

Diagnostic and treatment of structural heart illnesses can be extremely difficult due to the wide range of anomalies that can impair the structure and function of the heart. These disorders can cause abnormalities in hemodynamics and cardiac function by changing the dimensions, forms, or structural integrity of the heart's chambers, valves, septa, or large arteries. Depending on the underlying pathology and severity of the disease, structural heart disorders can present with a wide range of symptoms, such as dyspnea, chest discomfort, tiredness, palpitations, and syncope.

In the following sections, we will examine specific types of structural heart diseases, exploring their etiology, pathophysiology, clinical presentation, diagnostic approach, and therapeutic interventions. By gaining a deeper understanding of these conditions and their management principles, healthcare providers can effectively diagnose, treat, and optimize outcomes for patients with structural heart diseases. Let's start by discussing atrial and ventricular hypertrophy as we explore this.

ATRIAL AND VENTRICULAR HYPERTROPHY

Atrial and ventricular hypertrophy refer to an adaptive response of the heart to increased hemodynamic load, resulting in thickening or enlargement of the atrial and ventricular myocardium, respectively. These structural changes occur in response to conditions such as hypertension, valvular heart disease, or cardiomyopathies, and are characterized by alterations in cardiac chamber size, wall thickness, and function. Understanding the etiology, clinical manifestations, diagnostic evaluation, and management strategies for atrial and ventricular hypertrophy is essential for optimizing patient care and preventing complications associated with these conditions.

PATHOPHYSIOLOGY OF HYPERTROPHY

The heart's physiological responses to prolonged pressure or volume excess are represented as atrial and ventricular hypertrophy. The hypertrophic remodeling that occurs in cardiac cells in response to an increase in workload is typified by cellular expansion, increased protein synthesis, and changes in gene expression. Eccentric atrial and ventricular hypertrophy is typified by chamber dilatation and wall thinning, while concentric hypertrophy involves a consistent thickening of the myocardium.

CLINICAL MANIFESTATIONS

Atrial Hypertrophy: Atrial hypertrophy may manifest with symptoms such as palpitations, dyspnea on exertion, or atrial arrhythmias (e.g., atrial fibrillation). Physical examination findings may include an enlarged and hyperdynamic precordium, accentuated P waves on electrocardiography (ECG), and atrial enlargement on imaging studies such as echocardiography.

Ventricular Hypertrophy: Heart failure symptoms such as orthopnea, tiredness, dyspnea, or paroxysmal nocturnal dyspnea can be caused by ventricular hypertrophy. Physical examination findings may include significant QRS complexes with elevated voltage on the ECG, continuous and palpable left ventricular (LV) heave, and misplaced apical impulse.

DIAGNOSTIC EVALUATION

- **Electrocardiography (ECG):** ECG findings may reveal characteristic changes associated with atrial and ventricular hypertrophy, including P wave abnormalities (e.g., increased amplitude, duration, or dispersion) in atrial hypertrophy, and increased QRS voltage or repolarization abnormalities (e.g., ST-T wave changes) in ventricular hypertrophy.

- **Echocardiography:** The main imaging technique used to evaluate atrial and ventricular hypertrophy is transthoracic echocardiography, which offers comprehensive details on chamber size, wall thickness, and function. Doppler echocardiography may evaluate hemodynamics and valvular function, which helps in the assessment of related disorders such valvular heart disease.

- **Cardiac MRI:** Cardiac magnetic resonance imaging (MRI) may be used to further characterize atrial and ventricular hypertrophy, assess myocardial tissue characteristics, and evaluate for associated structural abnormalities or complications.

MANAGEMENT STRATEGIES

Management of atrial and ventricular hypertrophy focuses on addressing the underlying cause, optimizing hemodynamics, and preventing progression to heart failure or arrhythmias. Treatment may include antihypertensive medications, lifestyle modifications (e.g., sodium restriction, weight loss), and management of associated conditions such as valvular heart disease or cardiomyopathies. In select cases, surgical interventions such as valve repair or replacement, septal myectomy, or atrial fibrillation ablation may be indicated to alleviate symptoms and improve outcomes.

IMPORTANCE OF LONG-TERM MONITORING

Regular clinical evaluations, periodic imaging examinations, and careful observation of symptoms, cardiac function, and related comorbidities are necessary for the long-term therapy of atrial and ventricular hypertrophy. Healthcare practitioners can enhance the quality of life and optimize outcomes for patients with atrial and ventricular hypertrophy by employing evidence-based treatment techniques and offering continuous support and education.

CONGENITAL HEART DEFECTS

Congenital heart defects (CHDs) are structural abnormalities of the heart or great vessels that arise during fetal development and are present at birth. These defects can involve the heart's walls, valves, or blood vessels, leading to alterations in cardiac anatomy, function, and circulation. CHDs represent the most common type of birth defect, affecting approximately 1% of live births worldwide. Understanding the etiology, classification, clinical manifestations, diagnostic evaluation, and management strategies for congenital heart defects is essential for optimizing outcomes and improving quality of life for affected individuals.

ETIOLOGY AND PATHOPHYSIOLOGY

The etiology of congenital heart defects is multifactorial and may involve genetic, environmental, and developmental factors. Genetic abnormalities, such as chromosomal anomalies or gene mutations, play a significant role in CHD pathogenesis. Environmental factors, including maternal infections, exposure to teratogenic agents, maternal diabetes, or maternal substance abuse, can also contribute to the development of CHDs. During embryogenesis, errors in cardiac morphogenesis can result in structural malformations affecting cardiac septation, valve formation, or great vessel alignment, leading to the formation of congenital heart defects.

CLASSIFICATION OF CONGENITAL HEART DEFECTS

Congenital heart defects are classified based on their anatomical location, hemodynamic consequences, and pathophysiological features. Common types of CHDs include septal defects (e.g., atrial septal defect, ventricular septal defect), cyanotic heart defects (e.g., tetralogy of Fallot, transposition of the great arteries), obstructive lesions (e.g., coarctation of the aorta, pulmonary stenosis), and complex congenital anomalies (e.g., hypoplastic left heart syndrome). Classification systems such as the Bethesda classification or the International Pediatric and Congenital Cardiac Code (IPCCC) are used to standardize terminology and facilitate communication among healthcare providers.

CLINICAL MANIFESTATIONS

Clinical manifestations of congenital heart defects vary depending on the type, severity, and associated anomalies. Infants with critical CHDs may present with cyanosis, respiratory distress, feeding difficulties, poor weight gain, or signs of congestive heart failure shortly after birth. Less severe defects may manifest with murmur, palpitations, exercise intolerance, or recurrent respiratory infections. Some CHDs may remain asymptomatic until later in childhood or adulthood, particularly if hemodynamic consequences are minimal.

DIAGNOSTIC EVALUATION

- **Prenatal Diagnosis:** Congenital heart defects may be detected prenatally using fetal echocardiography, allowing for early identification and prenatal counseling.

- **Clinical Assessment:** Physical examination findings, including abnormal heart sounds, murmurs, cyanosis, or signs of heart failure, may raise suspicion for congenital heart defects.

- **Imaging Studies:** Echocardiography is the primary imaging modality for diagnosing and evaluating congenital heart defects, providing detailed information regarding cardiac anatomy, function, and hemodynamics. Additional imaging modalities, such as cardiac MRI or cardiac catheterization, may be indicated for further characterization or intervention planning.

MANAGEMENT STRATEGIES

Management of congenital heart defects depends on the type, severity, and associated complications. Treatment may include medical therapy, interventional procedures, or surgical repair. Medical management aims to optimize cardiac function, prevent complications, and improve quality of life. Interventional procedures, such as cardiac catheterization or balloon valvuloplasty, may be used to relieve obstructive lesions or close septal defects. Surgical repair is often necessary for complex defects or lesions that cannot be addressed by less invasive means. Long-term management involves regular follow-up, monitoring of cardiac function, and addressing associated comorbidities.

IMPORTANCE OF MULTIDISCIPLINARY CARE

The management of congenital heart defects requires a multidisciplinary approach involving pediatric cardiologists, cardiac surgeons, cardiac intensivists, nurses, and other healthcare providers. Collaboration among specialists is essential for comprehensive evaluation, treatment planning, perioperative care, and long-term follow-up of individuals with congenital heart defects. Additionally, patient education, psychosocial support, and advocacy for individuals and families affected by CHDs are integral components of holistic care delivery.

A wide range of anatomical anomalies known as congenital heart defects have important effects on afflicted individuals as well as their families. The prognosis of CHD patients has significantly improved thanks to developments in prenatal diagnosis, medicinal therapy, interventional procedures, and surgical methods. Healthcare professionals can effectively manage congenital heart abnormalities, optimize outcomes, and improve the quality of life for persons living with these disorders by implementing a patient-centered, multidisciplinary approach to care.

VALVULAR HEART DISEASES

Valvular heart diseases encompass a group of conditions characterized by abnormalities in the structure or function of the heart valves, leading to disturbances in blood flow, cardiac hemodynamics, and cardiac performance. These diseases can affect any of the four cardiac valves (aortic, mitral, pulmonary, and tricuspid) and may involve valve stenosis (narrowing), regurgitation (leakage), or a combination of both. Valvular heart diseases can result from congenital malformations, acquired disorders, degenerative changes, or inflammatory processes, and may lead to symptoms ranging from mild to severe, depending on the severity of valve dysfunction and associated hemodynamic consequences. Understanding the etiology, pathophysiology, clinical manifestations, diagnostic evaluation, and management strategies for valvular heart diseases is essential for providing comprehensive care to affected individuals.

ETIOLOGY AND PATHOPHYSIOLOGY

Valvular heart diseases can arise from various etiologies, including congenital abnormalities, degenerative changes, rheumatic fever, infective endocarditis, connective tissue disorders, or ischemic heart disease. These conditions can lead to alterations in valve structure, including leaflet thickening, calcification, fibrosis, or perforation, impairing valve function and causing valve stenosis or regurgitation. Chronic valve pathology may result in compensatory cardiac remodeling, chamber enlargement, or myocardial dysfunction, leading to heart failure or arrhythmias.

CLASSIFICATION OF VALVULAR HEART DISEASES

Valvular heart diseases are classified based on the affected valve, the nature of valve dysfunction (stenosis or regurgitation), and the underlying etiology. Common types of valvular heart diseases include aortic stenosis, mitral regurgitation, mitral stenosis, aortic regurgitation, tricuspid regurgitation, and pulmonary regurgitation. Valve lesions may be isolated or combined, and severity can range from mild to severe, based on the degree of valve obstruction or incompetence and associated hemodynamic consequences.

CLINICAL MANIFESTATIONS

Clinical manifestations of valvular heart diseases vary depending on the type, severity, and chronicity of valve dysfunction. Patients with valve stenosis may present with symptoms of exertional dyspnea, angina, syncope, or heart failure, reflecting increased pressure gradients across the stenotic valve and impaired cardiac output. In contrast, patients with valve regurgitation may present with symptoms of volume overload, including fatigue, palpitations, dyspnea on exertion, or peripheral edema, due to retrograde flow of blood into the preceding chamber during systole.

DIAGNOSTIC EVALUATION

- **Physical Examination:** Auscultation of heart sounds, including murmurs, clicks, or rubs, is essential for detecting valvular heart diseases and assessing their severity. Additional findings such as jugular venous distention, peripheral edema, or pulmonary crackles may provide clues to the presence of valvular dysfunction and associated hemodynamic abnormalities.

- **Echocardiography:** Transthoracic echocardiography is the primary imaging modality for diagnosing and evaluating valvular heart diseases, providing detailed information regarding valve morphology, function, and hemodynamics. Doppler echocardiography allows for assessment of flow velocities, gradients, and regurgitant volumes, aiding in the quantification of valve severity.

- **Cardiac Catheterization:** When echocardiographic results are unclear or inconsistent with the clinical presentation, invasive hemodynamic testing may be necessary to establish the diagnosis, evaluate the severity, and direct treatment choices.

MANAGEMENT STRATEGIES

The goals of valvular heart disease management are to reduce symptoms, enhance quality of life, and avoid consequences from valve malfunction. Depending on the kind, degree, and chronicity of valve pathology, treatment options may include medication, percutaneous or surgical valvuloplasty, or mechanical or bioprosthetic valve replacement. The degree of symptoms, the impact on hemodynamics, and the existence of comorbidities like endocarditis, arrhythmias, or heart failure all influence when to schedule intervention. In order to stop the disease's progression and enhance results, long-term care entails routine check-ups, valve function monitoring, and medication therapy modification.

IMPORTANCE OF COMPREHENSIVE CARE

Cardiologists, cardiac surgeons, cardiac imaging specialists, nurses, and other healthcare professionals must collaborate to manage valvular heart problems. For the purpose of providing valvular heart disease patients with an appropriate diagnosis, treatment planning, perioperative care, and long-term follow-up, collaboration amongst specialists is necessary. To further optimize results and enhance the quality of life for patients with valvular heart disorders, patient education, lifestyle changes, and adherence to medical therapy are essential elements of holistic care delivery.

CHAPTER SIX
Other Cardiac Conditions

In addition to the primary heart diseases that impact the myocardium, valves, or electrical conduction system, there are several other significant cardiac conditions that can profoundly affect an individual's health. These include disorders of the pericardium, inflammatory diseases of the heart muscle, infections of the endocardium, and even cardiac tumors, each presenting unique challenges in diagnosis and management. Since these illnesses frequently coexist with or mimic more common cardiovascular diseases, understanding them is essential for a holistic approach to cardiac care. This is because these conditions can complicate diagnosis and treatment plans.

Pericarditis refers to the inflammation of the pericardium, the fibrous sac surrounding the heart. This condition can cause sharp chest pain and other symptoms that may mimic myocardial infarction, necessitating distinct diagnostic and therapeutic approaches.

Myocarditis is the inflammation of the myocardium, the thick muscular layer of the heart wall. It can be caused by a variety of pathogens, immune responses, or toxic exposures, and is a common cause of sudden, unexpected heart failure in younger populations.

Endocarditis involves the inflammation of the inner lining of the heart chambers and valves, typically caused by infectious agents. It is a serious condition that can lead to severe valve damage and systemic complications if not promptly treated.

Cardiac tumors, though rare, can range from benign to highly malignant and may originate in the heart or spread from other parts of the body. Their presence can interfere with normal cardiac function and present with a wide array of symptoms.

This chapter looks into each of these conditions, discussing their pathophysiology, clinical presentation, diagnostic techniques, and current management practices. Healthcare professionals must comprehend these uncommon but serious cardiac disorders in order to treat patients more successfully and with better results.

PERICARDITIS

Pericarditis is an inflammation of the pericardium, the double-layered, sac-like structure surrounding the heart. This condition is characterized primarily by chest pain and other symptoms that can often mimic those of more serious cardiac issues, such as myocardial infarction. It is vital for healthcare providers to recognize and differentiate pericarditis to manage it effectively and prevent complications.

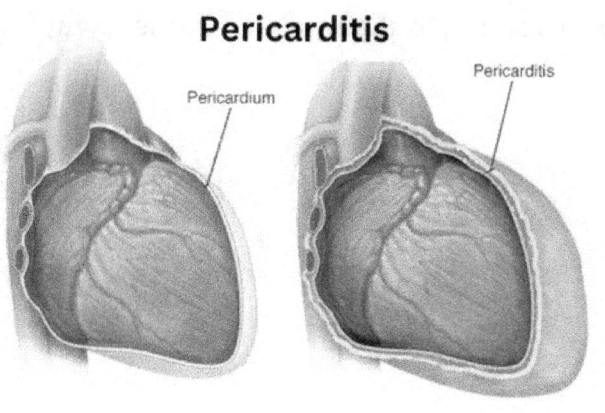

Fig 6.0: Pericarditis

ETIOLOGY AND PATHOPHYSIOLOGY

Pericarditis can be caused by a variety of factors, including viral infections (the most common cause), bacterial infections, fungal infections, autoimmune disorders, and following a heart attack or heart surgery. In many cases, however, the cause remains idiopathic. The inflammatory process typically results in an accumulation of fluid between the layers of the pericardium, leading to chest pain and other symptoms.

CLINICAL MANIFESTATIONS

- **Chest Pain:** Typically sharp and pleuritic in nature, the pain is usually felt behind the breastbone or in the left side of the chest. It may worsen with inhaling deeply, coughing, swallowing, or lying flat, and it often improves when sitting up or leaning forward.
- **Other Symptoms:** These may include fever, a feeling of weakness or fatigue, cough, palpitations, and occasionally, shortness of breath if the amount of fluid accumulating within the pericardium is sufficient to restrict heart function (cardiac tamponade).

DIAGNOSTIC EVALUATION

- **Electrocardiogram (ECG):** In the early stages of pericarditis, the ECG typically shows diffuse ST-segment elevation across multiple leads with a concave upward shape, which helps distinguish it from the changes seen in myocardial infarction.

- **Echocardiography:** This imaging technique is crucial for identifying pericardial effusion (fluid around the heart) and assessing its impact on cardiac function.

- **Blood Tests:** Elevated inflammatory markers such as C-reactive protein (CRP) and erythrocyte sedimentation rate (ESR), as well as markers of myocardial damage like troponin, may be helpful in the diagnosis.

- **Chest X-ray:** While not diagnostic for pericarditis itself, a chest X-ray can help exclude other causes of chest pain and detect pericardial calcification or an enlarged cardiac silhouette, suggesting a pericardial effusion.

MANAGEMENT STRATEGIES

- **Medical Management:** Treatment primarily involves managing pain and inflammation. Nonsteroidal anti-inflammatory drugs (NSAIDs) are the first-line treatment, often combined with colchicine to reduce inflammation and prevent recurrences. In severe cases, corticosteroids may be prescribed.

- **Monitoring and Follow-Up:** Patients with pericarditis should be monitored closely for signs of worsening condition, such as the development of cardiac tamponade, which is a life-threatening emergency requiring immediate intervention.

- **Pericardiocentesis:** In cases where cardiac tamponade threatens cardiac function, this procedure may be needed to remove excess fluid from the pericardial space.

PROGNOSIS AND COMPLICATIONS

Most cases of acute pericarditis have a good prognosis if treated promptly, though some may progress to chronic pericarditis or recurrent episodes. Complications can include constrictive pericarditis, a condition where the pericardium becomes thick and fibrous, restricting heart function and potentially leading to severe heart failure.

In order to properly diagnose and treat pericarditis, one must be aware of its many presentations and employ a comprehensive diagnostic process. This will enable fast initiation of appropriate therapy, preventing complications and guaranteeing the patient's best prognosis.

MYOCARDITIS

Myocarditis is an inflammation of the myocardium, the heart muscle itself. This condition can significantly impact heart function and is a notable cause of acute heart failure, particularly in young and otherwise healthy individuals. Myocarditis can vary widely in its presentation, ranging from mild symptoms to severe heart failure or sudden cardiac death.

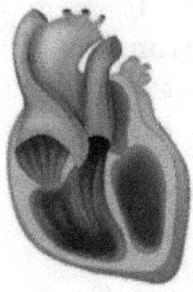
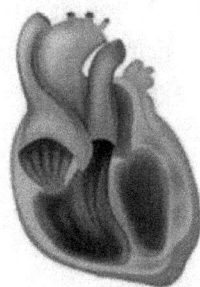

Fig 6.1: Myocarditis

ETIOLOGY AND PATHOPHYSIOLOGY

Enteroviruses (including the Coxsackie virus), adenoviruses, and parvovirus B19 are among the viruses that most frequently cause the inflammation in myocarditis. It may, however, also be the consequence of autoimmune disorders, bacterial or fungal infections, toxic reactions to specific drugs, or autoimmune diseases. A major reduction of cardiac function may result from the immune system's reaction to the infection, which frequently makes the damage to the heart muscle cells worse.

CLINICAL MANIFESTATIONS

- **Symptoms:** Patients with myocarditis often present with a variety of symptoms, including fatigue, shortness of breath, arrhythmias, and chest pain, which can mimic those of a heart attack. In severe cases, myocarditis can lead to heart failure, characterized by dyspnea, edema, and reduced exercise tolerance.
- **Physical Signs:** These could include murmurs, tachycardia (fast heartbeat), and symptoms of fluid overload such peripheral edema, pulmonary crackles, and jugular venous distention.

DIAGNOSTIC EVALUATION

- **Electrocardiogram (ECG):** ECG findings in myocarditis can be nonspecific but might include ST-segment and T-wave abnormalities, arrhythmias, or conduction abnormalities.

- **Blood Tests:** Elevated cardiac enzymes like troponin, which indicate myocardial damage, along with inflammatory markers such as CRP and ESR, are commonly observed.

- **Echocardiography:** This tool is crucial for evaluating left ventricular function and can help identify complications such as cardiac dilatation or dysfunction.

- **Cardiac MRI:** Magnetic resonance imaging (MRI) is particularly useful for diagnosing myocarditis. It can provide detailed images of the heart's structure and function, and it can specifically detect myocardial inflammation and necrosis.

- **Endomyocardial Biopsy:** Though invasive, this procedure is the gold standard for diagnosing myocarditis, allowing for direct tissue analysis.

MANAGEMENT STRATEGIES

- **Supportive Care:** Initial treatment focuses on managing symptoms, such as using diuretics for fluid overload and medications to control heart rate and blood pressure.

- **Specific Treatments:** Depending on the cause, treatments may include antiviral or antibacterial therapies, although their efficacy can vary. In cases where an autoimmune response is implicated, corticosteroids or other immunosuppressive agents may be considered.

- **Monitoring and Follow-Up:** Frequent follow-ups are necessary to monitor heart function and the progression or resolution of inflammation.

- **Lifestyle and Activity Modifications:** Patients are often advised to avoid competitive sports and strenuous activities during the acute phase of the disease to reduce the strain on the heart.

PROGNOSIS AND COMPLICATIONS

While many patients with myocarditis recover completely, some may develop chronic heart failure or dilated cardiomyopathy. In severe cases, myocarditis can lead to life-threatening arrhythmias or sudden cardiac death.

Myocarditis is still a difficult disorder because of its many manifestations and causes. Healthcare professionals must take into account myocarditis when treating patients who exhibit heart dysfunctional symptoms, particularly in younger patients without obvious coronary artery disease risk factors, as early detection and appropriate management are critical to improving outcomes.

ENDOCARDITIS

Endocarditis is a serious infection and inflammation of the inner lining of the heart chambers and valves (endocardium). It typically occurs when bacteria, fungi, or other microorganisms from another part of the body, such as the mouth, spread through the bloodstream and attach to damaged areas of the heart. If not treated promptly and effectively, endocarditis can damage or destroy heart valves and can lead to life-threatening complications.

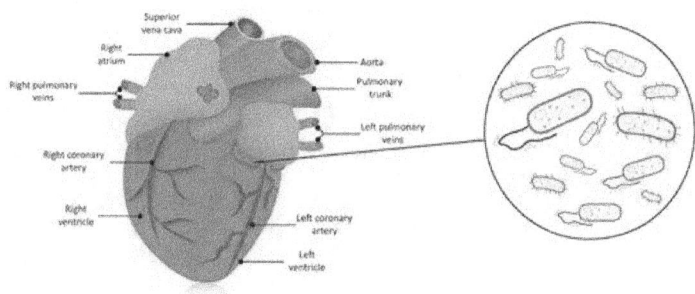

Fig 6.2: Endocarditis

ETIOLOGY AND PATHOPHYSIOLOGY

Bacterial infections, especially those caused by Enterococci, Streptococcus viridans, or Staphylococcus aureus, are the most frequent cause of endocarditis. A greater risk group includes those who have undergone heart valve replacements, have implanted devices, or have pre-existing cardiac problems. Because intravenous drug use frequently introduces bacteria into the circulation, there is also a large increase in risk.

CLINICAL MANIFESTATIONS

- **Fever:** This is the most common symptom, often accompanied by chills and night sweats.

- **Heart Murmurs:** New or changed heart murmurs are often detectable, reflecting valve damage caused by the infection.

- **Petechiae:** Small, pinpoint hemorrhages visible on the skin, inside the mouth, or on the whites of the eyes.

- **Osler's Nodes:** Painful, red, raised lesions found on the hands and feet.

- **Janeway Lesions:** Painless, flat, red spots seen on the palms and soles.

- **Other Symptoms:** Fatigue, weakness, weight loss, and joint pain.

DIAGNOSTIC EVALUATION

- **Blood Cultures:** Positive blood cultures are crucial for diagnosing endocarditis, helping identify the causative organism.

- **Echocardiogram:** An echocardiogram, particularly a transesophageal echocardiogram, is effective in visualizing the heart valves and any vegetations (masses of bacteria and cellular debris) present.

- **Complete Blood Count (CBC) and Other Labs:** Elevated white blood cell count, signs of anemia, and inflammatory markers are common.

- **Imaging Tests:** Additional imaging, such as CT or MRI, may be necessary to assess complications, especially in the brain or other organs.

MANAGEMENT STRATEGIES

- **Antimicrobial Therapy:** Prolonged and high-dose antibiotic therapy is usually required, often for several weeks to months, depending on the organism and severity of the infection. The treatment may start intravenously and switch to oral antibiotics as the condition improves.

- **Surgery:** Surgical intervention may be necessary to repair or replace damaged valves, remove large vegetation, or address complications like heart failure or abscess formation.

- **Prevention:** Patients at high risk, such as those with previous valve replacements or certain congenital heart defects, may require prophylactic antibiotics before dental or surgical procedures that could introduce bacteria into the bloodstream.

PROGNOSIS AND COMPLICATIONS

The death rate from endocarditis is high, particularly if treatment is postponed. Stroke, heart failure, valve perforation, and systemic emboli are possible complications. Aggressive therapy and early discovery are essential for better results.

The management of endocarditis requires a coordinated care approach involving cardiologists, infectious disease specialists, and often cardiac surgeons. Maintaining vigilance for this condition is crucial, especially in vulnerable populations, to ensure timely diagnosis and management.

CARDIAC TUMORS

Cardiac tumors, while rare, can either be primary (originating within the heart) or secondary (metastases from tumors located elsewhere in the body). These tumors can vary widely in their behavior, from benign to highly malignant, and their presence can significantly affect the heart's function and overall health outcomes.

ETIOLOGY AND CLASSIFICATION

- **Primary Cardiac Tumors:** They are not very common. The benign myxoma, which mostly affects the left atrium, is the most prevalent form. Other, less common forms include malignant sarcomas, lipomas, and fibroelastomas.

- **Secondary Cardiac Tumors:** These are more common than primary tumors and usually arise from metastasis of cancers from the lung, breast, melanoma, or lymphoma.

CLINICAL MANIFESTATIONS

Symptoms of cardiac tumors can mimic those of other heart conditions, making diagnosis challenging. They include:

- **Dyspnea:** Shortness of breath, often due to obstruction of blood flow or heart failure.

- **Palpitations:** Caused by arrhythmias that may develop as the tumor affects the heart's electrical system.

- **Chest Pain:** The tumor may induce angina-like pericardial pain or discomfort, depending on its size and location.

- **Systemic Symptoms:** Weight loss, fever, or changes in skin appearance can be seen in cases with malignant tumors.

- **Embolism:** Pieces of the tumor can break off and cause emboli, leading to strokes or peripheral embolization.

DIAGNOSTIC EVALUATION

- **Echocardiography:** A primary tool for visualizing the size, location, and hemodynamic impact of cardiac tumors.

- **MRI and CT Scans:** These provide detailed images that help in assessing the tumor's extent, its exact location, and involvement with surrounding structures.

- **Biopsy:** Although risky, a biopsy may be necessary to definitively diagnose the tumor type, particularly in suspected cases of malignancy.

MANAGEMENT STRATEGIES

- **Surgical Removal:** This is often the preferred treatment for primary cardiac tumors, especially benign ones like myxomas, to prevent complications such as embolism or obstruction.

- **Radiation and Chemotherapy:** These may be used for malignant tumors, depending on the type and extent of malignancy.

- **Monitoring and Supportive Care:** Regular follow-up imaging studies are necessary to monitor for recurrence or progression of the tumor. Supportive treatments, such as managing arrhythmias or heart failure, are also important.

PROGNOSIS AND COMPLICATIONS

The prognosis for patients with cardiac tumors varies significantly based on the type of tumor and whether it is benign or malignant. Benign tumors like myxomas, once removed, often have an excellent prognosis with low recurrence rates. Malignant tumors, however, may have a poor prognosis due to aggressive growth and the potential for metastasis.

Given their rarity, cardiac tumors require careful evaluation and management in specialized centers with experience in complex cardiac conditions. Early detection and appropriate intervention are crucial to managing potential complications and improving patient outcomes.

CHAPTER SEVEN
Pediatric Considerations

Electrocardiograms (ECGs) in pediatric patients present unique challenges and considerations that differ significantly from those in adults. Children's hearts are not just smaller versions of adult hearts; they exhibit different normal variants and developmental changes as they grow. It is crucial for healthcare providers to understand these differences to accurately interpret pediatric ECGs and diagnose any potential cardiac issues early on.

Children's ECGs can show normal variants that might be mistaken for pathological conditions if viewed without the context of pediatric norms. Conversely, certain abnormalities in pediatric ECGs might signal serious congenital or acquired heart diseases that require prompt attention and intervention. Recognizing these differences is essential for accurate diagnosis and management of pediatric cardiac conditions.

This chapter focuses on the normal variants in pediatric ECGs and the common abnormalities that healthcare providers may encounter. By understanding these aspects, practitioners can ensure better cardiac care for their younger patients and avoid misdiagnosis or unnecessary anxiety for both the patients and their families.

Age (years)	Respiratory rate (per minute)	Heart rate (per minute)
<1	30–40	110–160
1–2	25–35	100–150
2–5	25–30	95–140
5–12	20–25	80–120
>12	15–20	60–100

Fig 7.1: Respiratory and heart rates in children

NORMAL VARIANTS IN PEDIATRIC ECGS

Interpreting ECGs in pediatric patients requires a nuanced understanding of the physiological differences between children and adults. Children undergo significant developmental changes as they grow, and these changes are reflected in their ECGs. Recognizing the normal variants specific to different pediatric age groups is crucial to avoid misdiagnosis and unnecessary concern.

AGE-RELATED DIFFERENCES

Heart Rate:

- **Newborns:** Typically have higher heart rates ranging from 120 to 160 beats per minute (bpm).

- **Infants and Young Children:** The heart rate gradually decreases as the child grows, with infants around 100-160 bpm and young children 80-120 bpm.

- **Adolescents:** The heart rate approaches adult values, generally between 60-100 bpm.

Axis Deviation:

- **Right Axis Deviation:** Common in newborns and infants due to the relative dominance of the right ventricle at birth. It normalizes as the left ventricle becomes more dominant with growth.

- **Transition:** By age 1, the axis typically shifts towards a more neutral or leftward position.

QRS Complex:

- **Duration:** Shorter in children due to smaller heart size and faster conduction times.

- **Voltage:** Higher precordial R waves in the right chest leads (V1, V2) are common in infants due to right ventricular dominance. In older children and adolescents, the voltage may decrease as left ventricular dominance increases.

T-WAVE INVERSIONS:

- **Normal Inversions:** T-wave inversions in the right precordial leads (V1-V3) are normal in children up to adolescence. This is often referred to as a "juvenile T-wave pattern."

P-WAVE:

- **Amplitude and Duration:** The P-wave is generally smaller and shorter in duration in younger children compared to adults.

QT INTERVAL:

- **Rate-Dependent:** The QT interval varies with heart rate and is shorter in children. Corrected QT (QTc) values must be interpreted carefully using age-appropriate normal ranges.

- Specific Normal Variants

Sinus Arrhythmia:

- **Description:** A common finding where the heart rate varies with breathing (increases during inhalation and decreases during exhalation). It is a normal physiological response and usually more pronounced in children.
Short PR Interval:

- **Description:** A relatively short PR interval can be normal in children, reflecting faster conduction through the AV node.
- **Prominent U Waves:**

- **Description:** U waves may be more prominent in children, particularly in the precordial leads. This is generally considered a benign finding.

PRACTICAL EXAMPLES

Newborn ECG Example:

- **Findings:** Heart rate of 150 bpm, right axis deviation, tall R waves in V1, and T-wave inversion in V1-V3.

- **Interpretation:** Normal for age.

5-Year-Old ECG Example:

- **Findings:** Heart rate of 110 bpm, QRS duration of 70 ms, T-wave inversion in V1-V2.

- **Interpretation:** Normal for age, with juvenile T-wave pattern.

ADOLESCENT ECG EXAMPLE:

- **Findings:** Heart rate of 85 bpm, axis near 0°, normal QRS duration, positive T waves in precordial leads.
- **Interpretation:** Normal for age, approaching adult ECG characteristics.

Understanding these normal variants is essential for healthcare providers to accurately interpret pediatric ECGs and differentiate between benign findings and potential pathological conditions. This knowledge helps ensure that children receive appropriate care without unnecessary interventions or anxiety.

COMMON ABNORMALITIES IN PEDIATRIC ECGS

While normal variants are common in pediatric ECGs, certain abnormalities can indicate underlying cardiac conditions that require further investigation and management. Recognizing these abnormalities is crucial for timely diagnosis and treatment, which can significantly improve outcomes for pediatric patients.

CONGENITAL HEART DISEASE (CHD)

1. **Atrial Septal Defect (ASD):**

    - **ECG Findings:** Right axis deviation, right atrial enlargement, incomplete right bundle branch block (RBBB).

    - **Clinical Significance:** ASDs are common congenital defects that can lead to right heart volume overload if left untreated.

2. **Ventricular Septal Defect (VSD):**

    - **ECG Findings:** Left atrial enlargement, left ventricular hypertrophy (LVH) or right ventricular hypertrophy (RVH), depending on the size and location of the defect.

    - **Clinical Significance:** VSDs can cause increased pulmonary blood flow and pressure, potentially leading to heart failure and pulmonary hypertension.

3. **Tetralogy of Fallot:**

    - **ECG Findings:** Right axis deviation, RVH.

    - **Clinical Significance:** This is a complex congenital heart defect that requires surgical correction. It consists of four abnormalities: VSD, pulmonary stenosis, right ventricular hypertrophy, and an overriding aorta.

ARRHYTHMIAS

1. **Supraventricular Tachycardia (SVT):**

   - **ECG Findings:** Narrow QRS complexes, rapid heart rate typically over 180 bpm in infants and over 150 bpm in older children.

   - **Clinical Significance:** SVT is the most common pediatric arrhythmia. It can cause palpitations, dizziness, or heart failure if sustained for long periods.

2. **Wolff-Parkinson-White (WPW) Syndrome:**

   - **ECG Findings:** Short PR interval, delta wave (slurred upstroke of the QRS complex), wide QRS complex.

   - **Clinical Significance:** WPW is a pre-excitation syndrome that can lead to SVT and potentially life-threatening arrhythmias.

3. **Long QT Syndrome:**

   - **ECG Findings:** Prolonged QT interval adjusted for heart rate (QTc).

   - **Clinical Significance**: Long QT syndrome can predispose children to torsades de pointes and sudden cardiac death.

STRUCTURAL HEART DISEASE

1. **Hypertrophic Cardiomyopathy (HCM):**

   - **ECG Findings:** LVH, deep Q waves in the inferior and lateral leads, ST-segment, and T-wave abnormalities.

   - **Clinical Significance:** HCM is a genetic condition that can cause obstructive cardiomyopathy and is a leading cause of sudden cardiac death in young athletes.

2. **Dilated Cardiomyopathy (DCM):**

   - **ECG Findings:** LVH, left bundle branch block (LBBB), ST-segment, and T-wave abnormalities.

   - **Clinical Significance:** DCM leads to impaired systolic function and can result in heart failure and arrhythmias.

ELECTROLYTE IMBALANCE

1. **Hyperkalemia:**

   - **ECG Findings:** Tall, peaked T waves, wide QRS complex, flattened P waves.

   - **Clinical Significance:** Hyperkalemia can lead to life-threatening arrhythmias and requires immediate treatment.

2. **Hypokalemia:**

   - **ECG Findings:** Flattened or inverted T waves, U waves, ST-segment depression.

   - **Clinical Significance:** Severe hypokalemia can cause arrhythmias and muscle weakness.

3. **Hypocalcemia:**

   - **ECG Findings:** Prolonged QT interval.

   - **Clinical Significance:** Hypocalcemia can cause tetany, seizures, and cardiac arrhythmias.

INFLAMMATORY AND INFECTIOUS CONDITIONS

1. Myocarditis:

- **ECG Findings:** Sinus tachycardia, diffuse ST-segment and T-wave abnormalities, low voltage QRS complexes.

- **Clinical Significance:** Myocarditis, often due to viral infections, can cause heart failure and arrhythmias.

2. Pericarditis:

- **ECG Findings:** Diffuse ST-segment elevation, PR segment depression.

- **Clinical Significance:** Pericarditis can cause chest pain and, if associated with significant effusion, can lead to cardiac tamponade.

PRACTICAL EXAMPLES

1. ECG of a Child with SVT:
- **Findings:** Rapid heart rate of 200 bpm, narrow QRS complexes.
- **Interpretation:** Likely SVT; further evaluation and management are necessary.

2. ECG of a Teenager with HCM:
- **Findings:** Deep Q waves in leads II, III, and aVF, LVH, ST-segment changes.
- **Interpretation:** Consistent with hypertrophic cardiomyopathy; requires echocardiographic confirmation and genetic testing.

3. ECG of a Child with Tetralogy of Fallot:
- **Findings:** Right axis deviation, RVH.
- **Interpretation:** Suggestive of congenital heart disease; requires echocardiography for diagnosis.

Comprehending and recognizing these typical irregularities in pediatric electrocardiograms is imperative for prompt diagnosis and suitable handling of diverse cardiac ailments in children. For these young individuals, early intervention can dramatically enhance their prognosis and quality of life.

CONCLUSION AND CLINICAL APPLICATIONS

The diagnosis and treatment of a variety of cardiac disorders depend heavily on the ability to interpret ECGs, as this book has shown us to be. It is particularly important to take into account the distinct illness patterns and typical physiological variations in pediatric patients. Patient care and results can be greatly improved by having a solid understanding of ECG interpretation in addition to clinical expertise.

This final chapter synthesizes the key findings from each preceding chapter, highlights practical applications of ECG interpretation in clinical settings, and provides resources for further reading and continued education. Our goal is to equip healthcare providers with the knowledge and tools needed to confidently interpret ECGs, recognize critical cardiac conditions early, and implement effective treatment strategies.

SUMMARY OF KEY FINDINGS

Throughout this book, we have covered a wide array of topics related to the interpretation of ECGs and their applications in diagnosing cardiac conditions. Here are the key findings summarized for each major section:

UNDERSTANDING THE ROLE OF ECG IN CARDIAC DIAGNOSIS

- **Importance of ECGs:** ECGs are a fundamental diagnostic tool in cardiology, providing critical insights into heart rhythm, electrical activity, and underlying cardiac conditions.
- **Basic Interpretation Skills:** Mastery of ECG basics, such as understanding waveforms, intervals, and segments, is essential for accurate diagnosis.

MYOCARDIAL INFARCTION

- **STEMI and NSTEMI:** Differentiation between ST-segment elevation myocardial infarction (STEMI) and non-ST-segment elevation myocardial infarction (NSTEMI) is crucial for appropriate management and treatment.
- **ECG Markers:** Key markers like ST-segment elevation, Q-waves, and T-wave changes are indicative of myocardial injury and infarction.

ARRHYTHMIAS

- **Common Arrhythmias:** Recognition of arrhythmias such as atrial fibrillation, ventricular tachycardia, heart blocks, and supraventricular tachycardias is vital for timely intervention.
- **ECG Patterns:** Each arrhythmia presents with distinct ECG patterns that aid in diagnosis and treatment planning.

CARDIOMYOPATHIES

- **Types of Cardiomyopathies:** Hypertrophic, dilated, and restrictive cardiomyopathies have unique ECG features and clinical implications.
- **Impact on Heart Function:** Understanding the impact of these conditions on cardiac function guides therapeutic decisions.

ELECTROLYTE IMBALANCE

- **Electrolyte Effects on ECG:** Electrolyte imbalances, such as hyperkalemia, hypokalemia, and hypercalcemia, produce specific ECG changes that can be life-threatening if not corrected.
- **Importance of Monitoring:** Continuous monitoring and management of electrolyte levels are essential in patients with cardiac conditions.

STRUCTURAL HEART DISEASES

- **Hypertrophy and Defects:** Conditions like atrial and ventricular hypertrophy, congenital heart defects, and valvular diseases present with characteristic ECG findings.
- **Diagnosis and Management:** Accurate ECG interpretation helps in diagnosing these structural abnormalities and planning appropriate interventions.

OTHER CARDIAC CONDITIONS

- **Inflammatory Diseases:** Pericarditis, myocarditis, and endocarditis have distinct ECG features that aid in diagnosis and management.
- **Tumors:** Cardiac tumors, although rare, require careful ECG evaluation to detect and manage potential complications.

PEDIATRIC CONSIDERATIONS

- **Normal Variants:** Pediatric ECGs have age-specific normal variants that must be distinguished from pathological findings.
- **Common Abnormalities:** Recognizing common abnormalities in pediatric ECGs helps in the early detection and treatment of congenital and acquired heart diseases.

Rapid detection and reaction to ECG irregularities can save lives and enhance the standard of treatment for patients with heart problems. Using the information from these parts, healthcare professionals can enhance their ECG interpretation abilities, improving patient outcomes and diagnosis accuracy. A thorough understanding of both problematic and normal variants is essential for providing appropriate cardiac care, particularly in pediatric populations where variations in heart physiology may make diagnosis more difficult.

PRACTICAL APPLICATIONS IN CLINICAL SETTINGS

Interpreting ECGs accurately and efficiently in clinical settings is crucial for diagnosing and managing a wide range of cardiac conditions. Here are practical applications of the knowledge gained from this book in various clinical scenarios:

EMERGENCY DEPARTMENTS

Rapid Diagnosis of Myocardial Infarction:

- **STEMI Recognition:** Prompt identification of ST-segment elevation myocardial infarction (STEMI) using ECG criteria enables immediate reperfusion therapy, such as thrombolysis or percutaneous coronary intervention (PCI).

- **NSTEMI Management:** The diagnosis of non-ST-segment elevation myocardial infarction (NSTEMI) facilitates the planning of coronary angiography as well as the start of antiplatelet and anticoagulant medication.

ARRHYTHMIA IDENTIFICATION:

- **Atrial Fibrillation:** Quick identification of atrial fibrillation and initiation of rate control, rhythm control, and anticoagulation can prevent thromboembolic events.

- **Ventricular Tachycardia:** It is possible to save lives when ventricular tachycardia is identified and treated right away. This care may include antiarrhythmic medication treatment or possible defibrillation.

CARDIOLOGY CLINICS

Chronic Condition Management:

- **Heart Failure:** Regular ECG monitoring in patients with heart failure can detect arrhythmias or ischemic changes that require adjustments in therapy.
- **Cardiomyopathies:** ECGs are useful for monitoring disease progression in hypertrophic, dilated, and restrictive cardiomyopathies and guiding treatment plans.

ELECTROLYTE IMBALANCE MONITORING:

- **Hyperkalemia and Hypokalemia:** Routine ECGs in patients at risk for electrolyte imbalances, such as those on diuretics or with renal disease, can detect changes early, allowing for timely intervention.

PEDIATRICS

Congenital Heart Disease Screening:

- **Newborn Screening:** Early referral to pediatric cardiologists is made possible by early ECG screening, which can detect congenital cardiac problems such as atrial or ventricular septal defects in newborns and infants.

- **Arrhythmia Detection:** Pediatric ECG interpretation skills help in diagnosing arrhythmias like SVT or WPW syndrome, ensuring prompt treatment.

DEVELOPMENTAL FOLLOW-UP:

Normal Variants: While accurately recognizing pathological alterations that require follow-up, an understanding of normal pediatric ECG variants helps parents feel less anxious and avoids unnecessary studies.

INTENSIVE CARE UNITS (ICUS)

Continuous Monitoring:

- **Critical Patients:** Continuous ECG monitoring in critically ill patients allows for the rapid detection of life-threatening arrhythmias or ischemic events.

- **Post-Surgical Care:** In patients undergoing heart surgery, post-operative electrocardiogram monitoring can identify early signs of problems including myocardial infarction or arrhythmias.

COMPLEX CASE MANAGEMENT:

- **Multidisciplinary Approach:** Comprehensive care for complex cardiac cases is ensured by integrating ECG findings in a multidisciplinary team environment with other diagnostic technologies (such as MRI or echocardiography).

GENERAL PRACTICE

Routine Check-Ups:

- **Preventive Care:** Regular ECGs during routine check-ups for patients with risk factors (e.g., hypertension, diabetes) help in early detection of ischemic heart disease or arrhythmias.

- **Medication Monitoring:** ECGs are essential for monitoring the cardiac effects of certain medications, such as those prolonging the QT interval.

PATIENT EDUCATION:

- **Explaining Results:** Patient knowledge and adherence to treatment recommendations are improved when patients are informed about the results of their ECG.

- **Lifestyle Advice:** Using ECG results to illustrate the impact of lifestyle changes (such as smoking cessation or exercise) on heart health motivates patients towards healthier habits.

Applying practical ECG interpretation in a variety of clinical situations improves patient outcomes, increases diagnosis accuracy, and guarantees prompt cardiac condition intervention. Healthcare professionals may provide high-quality cardiac care in a variety of medical settings, including emergency rooms and general practices, by incorporating the concepts and information from this book.

FURTHER READING AND RESOURCES

To continue expanding your knowledge and stay updated with the latest developments in ECG interpretation and cardiac care, here are some recommended resources, including textbooks, online courses, websites, and journals.

TEXTBOOKS/ E-BOOKS

"Mastering ECG EKG Interpretation: A Comprehensive Guide for Beginners: ECG Interpretation Made Easy" by Joan Hampton
- A beginner-friendly book that simplifies ECG interpretation, making it accessible for students, healthcare professionals and, ideal for healthcare providers who interpret ECGs regularly.
Buy Now

"Electrocardiography in Emergency, Acute, and Critical Care" by Amal Mattu, MD
- A beginner-friendly book that simplifies ECG interpretation, making it accessible for students and healthcare professionals.**Buy Now**

"Goldberger's Clinical Electrocardiography: A Simplified Approach" by Ary L. Goldberger, Zachary D. Goldberger, and Alexei Shvilkin
- An excellent resource that provides practical approaches to ECG interpretation with numerous case studies and examples.**Buy Now**

ONLINE COURSES AND TUTORIALS

- Coursera – "ECG Assessment: An Introduction for Healthcare Providers"
- A free course that provides an introduction to ECG interpretation, suitable for beginners.

Medscape ECG Review
- A series of free tutorials and quizzes to test and improve your ECG interpretation skills.

ECG Academy
- Offers in-depth online courses ranging from basic to advanced ECG interpretation, created by Dr. Nicholas Tullo, a cardiologist.

VIDEO TRAINING

For those looking to enhance their ECG/EKG interpretation skills through visual and interactive learning, video training can be an excellent resource. Greenway Org offers a professional video training series designed to provide comprehensive instruction on ECG/EKG interpretation. This training is ideal for healthcare professionals at any stage of their career who want to deepen their understanding and improve their practical skills.

HOW TO OPT-IN FOR VIDEO TRAINING

You can access this exclusive video training offer by following these steps:

1. **Send an Email:**
   - Address your email to **greenwayorg1@gmail.com**.
   - Use the email subject line: **ECG/EKG Professional Video Training**.
2. **Exclusive Offer:**
   - Mention the **coupon code ECGEKG241** in your email to receive a special discount on the training series.
3. **What to Expect:**
   - The training series covers all aspects of ECG/EKG interpretation, from basic principles to advanced diagnostic techniques.
   - Content is delivered by experienced professionals and includes practical examples, case studies, and interactive components to enhance learning.
   - You will receive detailed instructions and access to high-quality video materials tailored to improve your proficiency in ECG/EKG interpretation.

Benefits of Video Training

- **Visual Learning:** Videos provide a dynamic way to learn ECG interpretation, making complex concepts easier to understand.
- **Interactive Components:** Engage with interactive exercises and quizzes to reinforce learning.

- **Practical Examples:** Real-world case studies and examples help bridge the gap between theory and practice.
- **Flexibility:** Learn at your own pace and revisit materials as needed to ensure mastery of the content.

Investing in video training can significantly enhance your ECG/EKG interpretation skills, providing you with a deeper understanding and greater confidence in clinical settings. Don't miss out on this opportunity to learn from professionals and gain access to high-quality training materials at a discounted price. Send your email today to greenwayorg1@gmail.com with the subject **ECG/EKG Professional Video Training** and use the coupon code **ECGEKG241** to take advantage of this exclusive offer.

Learn at your own pace and revisit materials as needed to ensure mastery of the content.

WEBSITES

Life in the Fast Lane (LITFL)

- A comprehensive online resource with tutorials, case studies, and quizzes on ECG interpretation.

ECG Library

- An extensive ECG database offering examples of normal and abnormal ECGs with detailed explanations.

American Heart Association (AHA)

- Provides guidelines, resources, and educational materials on ECG interpretation and cardiovascular care.

JOURNALS AND ARTICLES

Journal of Electrocardiology

- Publishes original research articles, reviews, and case reports on all aspects of electrocardiology.

Circulation: Arrhythmia and Electrophysiology

- A journal that covers the latest research and clinical practices related to cardiac arrhythmias and electrophysiology.

European Heart Journal – Acute Cardiovascular Care

- Offers articles on the latest advances in acute cardiac care, including ECG interpretation.

The Lancet: Cardiology

- Publishes cutting-edge research and reviews in cardiology, including studies on ECG interpretation and its clinical applications.

APPS AND TOOLS

QxMD Read
- A mobile app that curates the latest research articles based on your interests, including cardiology and ECG interpretation.

ECG Guide by QxMD
- An app that provides detailed ECG interpretation guides and clinical cases for learning on the go.

Figure 1
- A medical case-sharing app where healthcare professionals can share and discuss ECGs and other medical cases with peers worldwide.

Providing high-quality cardiac care requires staying current with new developments and always honing your ECG interpretation techniques. For both novice and seasoned healthcare professionals, the aforementioned resources give a plethora of knowledge and educational possibilities. You can increase patient outcomes by using these resources to broaden your knowledge, remain up to date on new discoveries, and so on.

ECG INTERPRETATION EXERCISES

EXERCISE 1

This exercise is designed to test your understanding of ECG interpretation through a practical scenario. Review the ECG tracing provided below and answer the corresponding questions. This will help you apply what you've learned and assess your ability to interpret ECG findings accurately.

ECG TRACING DESCRIPTION:

- **Rate:** Regular rhythm with a heart rate of about 75 beats per minute.
- Rhythm: Sinus rhythm.
- **P Wave:** Present before each QRS complex, normal morphology.
- **PR Interval:** 0.16 seconds.
- **QRS Complex:** Duration 0.10 seconds.
- **ST Segment:** Elevated in leads II, III, and aVF.
- **T Wave:** Inverted in leads II, III, and aVF.

QUESTIONS:

- What is the likely diagnosis based on the ECG tracing?
- Which area of the heart is most likely affected?
- What should be the immediate steps in managing this patient?

ANSWERS:

Likely Diagnosis:

- The ECG suggests ST-Segment Elevation Myocardial Infarction (STEMI).

Affected Area:

- The ST segment elevation in leads II, III, and aVF indicates that the inferior wall of the left ventricle is most likely affected.

Immediate Management Steps:

- Call for emergency help immediately (activate the emergency response system).
- Initiate monitoring of vital signs and establish IV access.
- Administer aspirin if not contraindicated, as it helps to prevent further clot formation.
- Prepare the patient for rapid transport to a facility with cardiac catheterization capabilities for potential percutaneous coronary intervention (PCI).
- Administer oxygen if there are signs of hypoxia or respiratory distress.
- Continuously monitor the ECG for any changes.

NOTE

This exercise serves as a practical application of your skills in ECG interpretation and underscores the critical importance of quick and accurate assessment in emergency cardiac care. Always remember, the precise interpretation of an ECG can be life-saving.

EXERCISE 2

This exercise will challenge you to apply your knowledge of ECG interpretation using another realistic scenario. Examine the ECG tracing information provided below and respond to the associated questions to solidify your understanding and diagnostic skills.

ECG TRACING DESCRIPTION:

- **Rate:** Fast, approximately 160 beats per minute.
- **Rhythm:** Regular.
- **P Wave:** Absent, with erratic spikes appearing.
- **PR Interval:** Not applicable due to absent P waves.
- **QRS Complex:** Narrow (<0.12 seconds).
- **ST Segment:** Not discernible.
- **T Wave:** Not clearly visible due to rapid rate.

QUESTIONS:

- What is the most probable diagnosis for this ECG tracing?
- What are the potential risks associated with this cardiac rhythm?
- What are the recommended treatment options for this condition?

ANSWERS:

Most Probable Diagnosis:

- This tracing is indicative of Atrial Fibrillation with a rapid ventricular response.

POTENTIAL RISKS:

- Atrial fibrillation, especially with a rapid rate, increases the risk of heart failure and stroke. The lack of effective atrial contraction leads to poor blood flow and can result in blood pooling and clot formation (thrombus), particularly in the atria.

RECOMMENDED TREATMENT OPTIONS:

- **Rate Control:** Medications such as beta-blockers or calcium channel blockers can be used to control the heart rate.
- **Rhythm Control:** Medications or electrical cardioversion may be considered to restore sinus rhythm.
- **Anticoagulation:** Depending on the patient's stroke risk, anticoagulants may be prescribed to prevent thromboembolic events.
- **Lifestyle Adjustments:** Addressing underlying causes and risk factors such as hypertension, obesity, and excessive alcohol intake.

NOTE

This exercise showcases the practical importance of identifying and appropriately treating atrial fibrillation to prevent long-term complications and improve patient outcomes. Your proficiency in reading and interpreting these signs on an ECG is crucial in clinical settings.

EXERCISE 3

This scenario offers a chance to further refine your skills in ECG interpretation. Examine the description of the ECG tracing below and answer the following questions to assess your analytical and diagnostic abilities.

ECG TRACING DESCRIPTION:

- **Rate:** Around 50 beats per minute.
- **Rhythm:** Regular.
- **P Wave:** Present, normal morphology, but not preceding every QRS complex.
- **PR Interval:** Variable; longer in cycles where a P wave precedes the QRS complex.
- **QRS Complex:** Normal duration (<0.12 seconds).
- **ST Segment:** Normal.
- **T Wave:** Normal.

QUESTIONS:

- What is the most likely diagnosis based on the ECG tracing?
- What is the physiological mechanism behind this condition?
- What are the potential treatment options or management strategies for this condition?

ANSWERS:

Most Likely Diagnosis:

- The ECG suggests Second-Degree AV Block, Type II (Mobitz II).

Physiological Mechanism:

- This type of block occurs when some of the electrical impulses from the atria are not conducted to the ventricles. In Mobitz II, the PR interval of conducted beats is constant, but some impulses fail to result in ventricular contraction, which is typically more dangerous than Type I and can be a precursor to a complete heart block.

POTENTIAL TREATMENT OPTIONS OR MANAGEMENT STRATEGIES:

- **Monitoring:** Close observation with continuous ECG monitoring to detect any progression to a more severe block.
- **Pacemaker:** If the patient shows signs of hemodynamic instability or if the block worsens, implantation of a pacemaker may be necessary.
- **Avoidance of Certain Medications:** Medications that can further impair AV conduction (like certain beta-blockers and calcium channel blockers) should be used cautiously or avoided.
- **Management of Underlying Conditions:** Addressing any underlying heart disease or conditions contributing to the AV block.

NOTE

This exercise is designed to test your ability to recognize more complex cardiac rhythms and understand their clinical implications, which are essential skills in the management of cardiac patients.

CONCLUSION

This book has aimed to provide a comprehensive guide to ECG/EKG interpretation, covering a wide range of cardiac conditions and their manifestations on ECG tracings. From the foundational principles of ECG interpretation to the nuances of recognizing specific cardiac conditions, each chapter has been designed to enhance your understanding and application of this essential diagnostic tool.

In the first chapters, we explored the basics of ECG interpretation, laying the groundwork for recognizing normal and abnormal patterns. We then went further into specific cardiac conditions, such as myocardial infarctions, arrhythmias, cardiomyopathies, and structural heart diseases, illustrating how each presents on an ECG. Special considerations for pediatric patients and the impact of electrolyte imbalances on ECG readings were also discussed, highlighting the importance of context in interpreting ECGs accurately.

Practical excersies in clinical settings emphasized how this knowledge translates into real-world scenarios, ensuring that healthcare providers can promptly and effectively diagnose and manage cardiac conditions.

By mastering ECG/EKG interpretation, you are better equipped to make informed decisions, improve patient outcomes, and advance your clinical expertise. This skill is vital across various medical fields, from emergency departments to specialized cardiology clinics, and is a cornerstone of effective cardiac care.

We hope this book has not only expanded your knowledge

but also inspired confidence in your ability to interpret ECGs. Continue to practice, learn, and stay updated with the latest advancements in cardiology. Your dedication to understanding and applying ECG interpretation will make a significant difference in the lives of your patients. Thank you for embarking on this journey with us, and we wish you continued success in your medical career.

ABOUT THE AUTHOR

Dr. Joan Hampton, a successful cardiologist with decades of experience, is renowned for her ability to elucidate the electrical symphony of the heart. Her engaging teaching style has earned her recognition as a dynamic and inclusive educator, empowering students in their journey to master ECG and EKG interpretation. One of her notable works is "Mastering ECG/EKG Interpretation: A Comprehensive Guide for Beginners," which simplifies ECG interpretation for readers at all levels.

Dr. Hampton combines her clinical expertise with a passion for teaching, ensuring that readers, regardless of their background, can confidently navigate the complex language of the heart.

DR JOAN HAMPTON

THE END

www.ingramcontent.com/pod-product-compliance
Lightning Source LLC
Chambersburg PA
CBHW071916210526
45479CB00002B/441